CLINICAL CLERKSHIPS

PETER WAYS
JOHN D. ENGEL
PETER FINKELSTEIN

CLINICAL CLERKSHIPS

The
Heart of
Professional
Development

Sage Publications, Inc.
International Educational and Professional Publisher
Thousand Oaks ▪ London ▪ New Delhi

"Death Psalm: O Lord of Mysteries" by Denise Levertov, from *Life in the Forest,* copyright © 1978 by Denise Levertov. Reprinted by permission of New Directions Publishing Corp.

"Gaudeamus Igitur" reprinted by permission of Louisiana State University Press from *Renaming the Streets: Poems,* by John Stone. Copyright © 1985 by John Stone.

For information:

Sage Publications, Inc.
2455 Teller Road
Thousand Oaks, California 91320
E-mail: order@sagepub.com

Sage Publications Ltd.
6 Bonhill Street
London EC2A 4PU
United Kingdom

Sage Publications India Pvt. Ltd.
M-32 Market
Greater Kailash I
New Delhi 110 048 India

Printed in the United States of America

Library of Congress Cataloging-in-Publication Data

Ways, Peter, 1928–
Clinical Clerkships: The Heart of Professional Development / by Peter Ways,
    John Engel, and Peter Finkelstein.
       p. cm. — (Surviving medical school)
    Includes bibliographical references and index.
    ISBN 0-7619-1831-0 (pbk.: acid-free paper)
    1. Clinical clerkship. I. Engel, John. II. Finkelstein, Peter. III.
Title. IV. Series.
    R839 .W39 2000
    610'.71'55—dc21   00-008075

This book is printed on acid-free paper.

00   01   02   03   04   05   06   7   6   5   4   3   2   1

Acquisition Editor:	Rolf Janke
Editorial Assistant:	Heidi van Middlesworth
Production Editor:	Sanford Robinson
Copy Editor:	Linda Gray
Editorial Assistant:	Cindy Bear
Typesetter:	Tina Hill
Indexer:	Molly Hall
Cover Designer:	Michelle Lee

Contents

Foreword

For decades, clinical training for medical students took place on the wards of teaching hospitals. Now, many former full-time faculty members are in private practice and teach at community hospitals, outpatient clinics, or their private offices. Patients with rare and esoteric conditions, once prized as teaching subjects, may be seen less often and those with common illnesses more often. Physicians, new and old, must learn to care for patients expertly and efficiently within the constraints of the managed-care system.

Some things, however, have not changed. The basic clinical clerkships of medicine, surgery, OB-GYN, pediatrics, psychiatry, and family medicine still take place in teaching hospitals and continue to require long hours, insufficient sleep, and emotional hardiness. A dehumanizing hierarchy still demands mastery of technical facts and often excludes or minimizes the affective aspects of medicine.

Clinical work continues to be not only a defining *professional* experience but a salient *life* experience as well, one that can bring about major changes in one's style of work, perspectives, and values. The professionalization that occurs during the clinical rotations sometimes comes at the expense of emotional and spiritual health. Furthermore, students or faculty rarely perceive this deficiency.

This superb book is written by three of the nation's leading medical educators. While at Michigan State University's College of Human Medicine, Peter O. Ways, MD, developed the first problem-based learning approach now used in preclinical training in many U.S. medical schools. Later, at the University of Illinois—Chicago, he was commissioned by the Association of American Medical Colleges (AAMC) to organize and manage an interview study of student reactions to the first two years of medical school. Since the mid-1980s, Dr. Ways has worked in addiction medicine and has continued to champion health prevention and maintenance.

John D. Engel, PhD, Executive Associate Dean at Northeastern Ohio University College of Medicine, is responsible for the school's education programs and evaluative efforts. As a pioneer in the definition and use of qualitative research paradigms in medical education, Dr. Engel directed a qualitative study (the first time these three authors collaborated) of students during their clinical clerkships, observing over 500 hours of clerkship activities. He developed the University of Delaware-Jefferson Medical College integrated program, where students are accepted for premed studies with the understanding that if they complete their courses satisfactorily, medical school admission will follow without further application.

Peter Finkelstein, MD, a psychiatrist in private practice, has acted as preceptor for numerous psychiatry residents in the Stanford Medical School program. While a resident at Stanford, Dr. Finkelstein conducted a five-year study of the anatomy lab experience. He spent 300 hours directly observing medical student affect, reactions, and adaptations to working with human cadavers. He found a causative connection between students' preclinical experiences and the ways they function in their clinical rotations the last two years of medical school.

These distinguished authors provide a wealth of important and interesting information and ideas to make your clinical clerkships satisfying, productive, and potentially healthier.

—Robert Holman Coombs
Professor of Biobehavioral Sciences, UCLA School of Medicine
Series Editor

NOTE: Throughout the text, *key points* appear in italics, and **key behaviors** appear in boldface.

Dedication

With deep respect and gratitude we dedicate this book to our primary mentors Andrew D. Hunt, MD, and Hilliard Jason, MD (Dr. Ways), Anthony LaDuca, PhD, and Betty Risley, PhD. (Dr. Engel), and Tom Johnson, MD (Dr. Finkelstein). They have enlivened our thinking, honored our feelings, nurtured our talent, and encouraged risks.

This work is also dedicated to the late Marianne (Tracy) Paget, sociologist, philosopher, and dear friend. Tracy probed the institutions and rituals of medicine with deep criticism while holding its practitioners and students in respect and love.

We also honor our students, past and present, who have endured remarkable trials yet emerged as sensitive and caring physicians. They have triumphed despite a traditional, often archaic educational milieu that can objectify its students, sever head from heart, engender mind-numbing exhaustion, and fail to provide constancy of focus on quality patient care and service.

Acknowledgments

Our former colleagues in the phenomenologic/anthropologic study of clerkships, Constance Filling, Karen Johnson, Richard Foley, and Larry LaPalio, helped substantially to define the nature and salient issues of the implicit curriculum. We owe them our deepest thanks. We are also particularly grateful to Eric Cassell for his landmark work on suffering, and to Allen Enelow and Scott Swisher, who wrote so definitively and helpfully about the interview process in medicine. Lura Pethtel, John Foglio, Howard Brody, Barry Rosen, and Heather, Carol, Martha, and Peter F. Ways, have all validated and stregthened our belief in the necessity to explore and access the spiritual dimension as a requisite part of integrated, whole-person care.

Our greatest editorial debt is to Brigid Ways Marcuse, a lively and perspicacious critic of both the health care system and of educational process. Ms. Marcuse spent untold hours critiquing the ideas and syntax of the manuscript. As a result, the product is unquestionably clearer, truer, and more reader friendly. We are also extremely grateful to Carol Coombs and to Gretchen Gundrum (Ways), who read earlier versions and offered many important suggestions for change and emphasis. Larry Hulbert and David Zucker offered valuable criticism in selected areas and repeatedly boosted our morale. Our thanks also to Gillen Nagy who spent many patient and skillful hours reprocessing the manuscript, and to Isaac Dockter and Zach Gundrum who created some of our figures and tables.

Last, but far from least, we thank Dr. Robert Coombs, who believed in our ability to effectively illuminate the clinical learning experience, and to Sage Publications for investing in his judgement. At Sage, Heidi van Middlesworth made valuable and important suggestions for shortening the manuscript, and Linda Gray, was an empathetic and skillful copy editor—her surgery was virtually painless! Sanford Robinson and Rolf Janke were patient and graceful in easing the manuscript through editing, formatting, and publication to achieve its metamorphosis as a real book.

Part I

Preparation and Expectations:
The Lay of the Land

1 Clerkships and the Ideal Physician

What any era considers the ideal physician reflects an amalgam of the demands made by the reigning theory of medicine, the social forces acting on doctors and sick persons, and the general social attitudes toward persons and their relations with each other.

—*Eric Cassell (1991, p. ix)*

Clinical clerkships are the heart and soul of undergraduate medical education and the true beginning of physicianhood. They are the learning vehicle for two of the four most formative years (M-3, M-4, PGY-1, PGY-2)[1] during which the patterns, values, and standards of your professional life are seeded and mature. You evolve into the kind of person and doctor that you will truly be. *Medicine is demanding and compelling. Patterns that you adopt or reinforce during training can profoundly affect many other aspects of your life.*

So why this book on clerkships? Your authors have broad experience in medical education. We have been students, residents, researchers, teachers, administrators, curriculum innovators, student advocates, and critics of the system. We have collaborated in teaching and research across the entire span of medical school, residency, and private practice. Our most extensive and privileged experience has been in the conduct and study of clinical education. We view medicine and medical education through a wider, more revealing lens than most faculty and administrators. Other books designed to guide and support students through the clerkships of the third and fourth year describe the work mostly as if it demands only cognitive and psychomotor skills and the

4 PREPARATION AND EXPECTATIONS

ability to get along with a variety of people. They discuss too briefly or not at all, a set of phenomena we term *the hidden or implicit (unstated) curriculum.* Scant attention is paid to the personal depletion (exhaustion, anxiety, depression), diminished emotional responsiveness, threat to intellectual vitality, endangered relationships, and work habits and discipline required to become a good physician. Little recognition is given to helping students deal with the emotional stresses of patient care, including those evoked by degradation and end-of-life issues. Finally, *there is a negligent lack of attention to suffering* as both a ubiquitous dimension of illness (Cassell, 1991) and as a personal experience for students and residents themselves.

These pages sculpt and nuance a characterization of the third and fourth years. We extend an invitation to critically engage with your education, reflect on your experiences, and prepare to be changed by them. Our overriding goal is *to expand your view of medical education and doctoring to include the implicit (unstated) curriculum, thus preparing you for difficulties not commonly discussed by deans, educators, practitioners, professors, or lab assistants but that are, unmistakably, an integral part of being a student and a doctor.* We intend more than description. This book will help with the how-to-do-it, but more important, it is written to stimulate discovery, growth, appropriate vulnerability, tolerance for uncertainty, and risk taking. It can help you emerge from clerkships and residency as a complete person, with a fuller appreciation of yourself, with balance in your life, and still retaining the willingness to work with your patients as whole, complex people. Our intent is to help you **be** as well as **do.**

Part I discusses expectations, faculty, discipline, and some practical aspects of getting ready for your initial major clerkships. Part II is devoted to the actual work you will be involved in, with chapters on honoring the patient, communication, the patient appraisal, rounds and teamwork, working with the family, and evaluation. In Part III, the implicit or hidden material and expectations are laid out: exhaustion, anxiety, depression, death, diminished emotional responsiveness, suffering, and loss of intellectual vitality. Part IV outlines the self-care that will help you get through medical school with a minimum of damage.

As reflected in our experience and in the most sensitive of writing about the professions (Carlson & Shield, 1989; Reynolds & Stone, 1991, 1995), medicine is a place of unusual privilege, with surfeits of satisfaction, hard work, ambiguity, sadness, frustration, and joy. There is abundant opportunity to help others, both in the diagnosis and management of their problems and in the relief of suffering. We invite you to use these pages as a sensitizing primer to understand your behavior and reactions to various situations. We hope they will contribute positively to your development as truly mature and compassionate physicians.

The Ideal Physician

What qualities do ideal physicians exhibit? Here is our answer: First and foremost, they have the skills and knowledge necessary to provide safe ("do no harm"), effective care to their patients. They can do excellent work in health maintenance and prevention, as well as in acute and chronic illness. With colleagues in conference and through reading, they explore critical aspects of patient care, frame important questions about the diagnostic and treatment issues at hand, and ferret out the impact that illness and suffering will have on the patient and family, as well as any family dynamics that may influence healing.

Our ideal physicians are scrupulously honest, particularly about themselves. They are good self-evaluators—aware of both their strengths and weaknesses. They are patient, thorough, humble, disciplined, and sensitive; they cherish enjoyment in all aspects of life. They live what they encourage and advise for their patients—successfully balancing their work and personal lives.

These physicians do not detour around pain and suffering but acknowledge them deeply and play a part in relieving them. They neither shield themselves from nor belittle their own importance to patients by being perfunctory, arrogant, presumptuous, disinterested (too busy), or insincere. We hope for women and men who can be attentive, empathetic, genuine, and helpful to most of their patients. They experience a full repertoire of feelings and choose to express them in ways that will benefit themselves, their patients, friends, and families.

We hope you will be able to say, "I don't know" as a responsible, professional action that leads, without shame, to the necessary remediation. We want you to accept that medicine is a profession in which errors are common and that to carry unresolved guilt or shame about them is to compound their impact. Be able to admit and talk about your errors—to say, "I was wrong," "I made a mistake." We hope you can react as Hilfiker (1991) suggests: "Shown our mistakes and forgiven them, we can grow, perhaps in some small way become better people. Mistakes understood in this way are a process, a way we connect with one another and with our deepest selves" (p. 379).

We hope that with Dr. William Carlos Williams you will believe, "Whole lives are spent in the treacherous affairs of daily events without even approaching the great sights that I see every day" (Williams, 1991, p. 75). **It is our hope that you will endeavor to see and interact with patients not as fragments in your day, not as repositories for disease or injury, not in any of the other myriad ways we can dehumanize or objectify patients but as whole people who are suffering, often afraid, and magnificent.**

The organization and financial structuring of medical practice are changing. At one level, these changes do not seem congruent with our vision. Be aware of this, but place it in broad historical perspective. The practice of medicine has always been bound by social and economic conditions, but as they relate to the essence of medicine, these conditions are not deterministic. *When all is said and done, the essence of medical practice—"Medicine"—will always be a transaction of intimacy between two human beings.*

Note

1. M-3 and M-4 refer to the third and fourth years of medical school. PGY-1 and PGY-2 refer to the first and second postgraduate years.

2 Expectations and Realities

As a neophyte medical student, you fantasized about being an important member of the patient care team—making rounds, working with patients, becoming, at last, a real doctor. The abundant lore associated with clerkships shaped your expectations. Some clerkships are known for a consistently rich and varied experience, respect for students, and excellent teaching. They are coveted. More commonly, you will have mixed expectations, focusing primarily on the variety of patients and the quality of teaching. You may fear assignment to certain faculty members because they teach poorly or are said to be demanding, forceful, racist, or sexist. Some nurses are helpful and nurturing; others, overbearing. Most of the house staff will be sympathetic and instructive but there will be stories about one or two who are lazy or controlling. Some hospitals and clerkships are not receptive to students; patients are not adequately briefed about the teaching hospital milieu and are surprised, and sometimes hostile, to be seen and evaluated by a medical student.

Whatever your preconceptions—and they will differ for you and your classmates—they will meld into a fantasy preview that may seem pleasurable, neutral, or alas, ominous.

Activity: In the following spaces, list your most prominent expectations for your next major specialty clerkship.

Then consider the following:

What do I most want to get out of it?

_____

What do I think will be most difficult about it?

_____

What am I most anxious about?

_____

What quality of teaching do I expect?

_____

Discuss your responses with a colleague or friend. Part way through the clerkship, look at them again. How does reality measure up?

Advice

1. It works best to minimize your preconceptions about patients, the nature of the experience, and the quality of the teaching. This will

   a. give you more incentive to create a rewarding situation for yourself;
   b. keep you open to a greater range of possibilities;
   c. minimize disappointment and frustration.

2. Remember that you are the most important variable in your own learning experience. You have more control than anyone over the quality of the experience and how much you learn. *Even in a poor learning environment, it is possible to salvage a positive experience.*

Basic Realities

Clerkships will vary. The staffing and duration of the clerkship will be one of several patterns (see Table 2.1). All will include an attending physician; many will have residents. Their lengths vary.

Table 2.1   Some Characteristics of Clerkships

Type of Clerkship	Faculty	Residents[a]/ Fellows	Duration	Outpatient/ Inpatient
Major specialty	General or subspecialty attendings[b]	Residents or subspecialty fellows (consultations)	6 weeks-3 months	Mostly inpatient but family medicine is outpatient
Subspecialty (e.g., cardiology; ear, nose, throat)	Subspecialty attendings	Subspecialty fellows or residents	1 week-4 weeks	Inpatient and outpatient
Critical care	Attendings	Subspecialty fellows or residents	1 week-2 months	Medical and surgical intensive care unit (IP), emergency room (OP)
PCCC[c]	General internal medicine and family medicine attendings	Residents	Once or more a week for 1-3 years	Outpatient

a. In a university system, all inpatient and most outpatient clerkships will have residents assigned.
b. Attending physicians.
c. Primary care continuity clerkship.

Differences in Outpatient and Inpatient Clerkships

Hospital-Based Inpatient Clerkships. You will work on the medical, surgical, pediatric, psychiatric, and OB-GYN services. Some will have both critical care and standard care units. You will probably be assigned to one or the other, although your time may be divided. Hospital patients are generally sicker, and their care is more intense than outpatients; they are more likely to die. Critical care and the ER are always intense and busy.

Outpatient Clerkships. On the typical outpatient clerkship, your patients have acute self-limited disease and/or chronic illness. You may see some patients two or more times during the clerkship. They may remain quite stable (noninsulin-dependent diabetes, rheumatoid arthritis), exhibit slow evolution of their problem, or have dramatic changes (diabetic ketoacidosis, or an acute gouty joint). Most outpatients are not as sick as inpatients. Generally, you spend less time with each patient, and there is less "scut" work (see glossary) than in the hospital. Stress levels depend on the frequency of scheduling and how many unscheduled walk-ins are seen.

Primary Care Continuity Clerkship (PCCC). This clerkship is an important exception to the one-clerkship-at-a-time pattern. In the typical PCCC, students go to clinic a half day to a full day a week throughout the third and/or the fourth year. Usually, you will attend the PCCC session while assigned to other clerkships. This may feel interruptive, but it reflects real life in practice. Its value lies in seeing some patients repeatedly over time, following their response to certain treatment programs, and observing the natural history of their illness. This clerkship is staffed by family practice or internal medicine.

Private Contrasted With Nonprivate Teaching Patients

Although often blurred, this distinction is important because private patients may not want to be seen by medical students. Most private patients want their own doctors to approve and supervise everything. With private patients, there may be fewer opportunities to learn procedures and write orders. How the attending introduces you to patients is important. "This is Steve Jones, a medical student and a colleague. He will work with you under my close supervision." **Make sure your attending tells his or her private patients that you, a medical student, will do their history and physical exam and about any other responsibilities you will have.**

Reasonable Expectations and Potential Surprises

When you actually arrive on the service, your own reality will unfold. Much of what you expect will be accurate and well-founded:

- Most of the pathology will fall within the purview of the specialty or subspecialty of the clerkship.

- The major specialty clerkships (internal medicine, surgery, pediatrics, family medicine, OB-GYN, and psychiatry) will be considerably longer than the others.
- Hours will be long.
- Rounds are important, although sometimes tedious.
- It is essential to do the scut work.
- Most of your work with patients will be highly gratifying (and at times hectic, difficult, frustrating, and/or emotionally painful).
- If you write orders, they must be countersigned by a house officer or an attending physician.
- You will see a variety of *illnesses* but may see several people with the same or similar *disease* diagnoses (see glossary).

However, some of your expectations may prove to be off target. You may, for example, *expect* that night call will consistently be an "exhausting drag" but *find* that being the only student on call with residents when there is less scheduled activity is very profitable. There is more time to talk with patients or chat over coffee with your resident. The radiologist on-call may spend extra time going over films with you. There is greater opportunity to be the first to interview and examine new admissions. Many nights are exhilarating.

Or you may expect (especially early in the house staff year) that the house staff will "hog" the procedures only to find this group very willing to share the riches.

You may have trepidation about being called "Doctor" when you are definitely not one, but to your great relief, your attending introduces you as, "Edward Halibut, our new student physician," or "our new third-year medical student."

You may expect that knowledge is the defining parameter on a clerkship: To do well, you will need to know all about the diseases of the specialty involved. On most clerkships, *you will find that knowledge is definitely important but that doing well involves a lot more than knowing facts and concepts.* It involves learning and perfecting the skills of interviewing/history-taking and physical examination. It definitely involves getting your work done promptly and proficiently.

You may be worried that you won't have enough responsibility, and then find yourself with more responsibility than you're comfortable with. **If you feel too much responsibility, don't be afraid to say so.** Nothing feels worse than being in over your head, with its attendant risk of drowning! *Students who know and heed their own limits are respected.*

Hidden and Ignored Realities:
The Implicit (Unstated) Curriculum

> **Warning!** Catalogue statements and opinions of colleagues never tell the whole story of a clerkship. In most phases of medical school, the explicit curricular outline describes what will happen and what is expected, but almost invariably, another set of expectations and experiences go unstated.

The Implicit Curriculum Revealed

The implicit curriculum is made up of many and varied emotionally draining events (e.g., sad, fearful, repugnant, frightening) that inevitably occur in medicine. How faculty expect students to behave in response to these events is often unstated as well. Certain aspects of the work environment also contribute. Unfortunately, while of utmost importance, this other cirriculum is seldom discussed with students by faculty. This is a serious deficiency in educational practice.

Impact of the Implicit Curriculum on Psyche and Spirit

The most important aspect of the unstated curriculum is its profound impact on your psyche and spirit. These injuries are compounded by constraints (also part of the implicit curriculum) against responding to them in healthy ways. Dr. Ways tells the following story:

Pediatrics, my first major clinical clerkship, was in a prestigious hospital that cared well for very sick children. Two classmates and I showed up at 7:30 a.m. the first day. We were each immediately assigned four patients. I was led to Ned's crib by a nurse who said, "Ned is five and has widespread neuroblastoma, a multicentric neurological tumor. He is not an easy patient to be with or take care of." Despite her warning, I was totally unprepared for the grotesque lad I met. He was a miniature Quasimoto—the hunchback of Notre Dame. Several orange- to grapefruit-sized tumor masses stuck out of his head, back, and abdomen. That Ned could move around with them, or even still be alive, seemed impossible. I wished he was semicomatose or unable to talk so that I wouldn't have to communicate with such a "pitiful" (my feeling) creature, but he was wide awake and lying on his side. I was afraid to touch him; such effervescent tumors must be contagious. The nurse introduced us, then departed, leaving me to talk with Ned and find a vein intact enough to draw some blood. He was receiving harsh chemicals to forestall the tumor's progress, and his lab data needed to be carefully monitored. I was at ease taking blood from adults but had never touched a sick child. Ned's arms were a mass of bruises and clotted veins—especially at the elbow and wrist where blood had been drawn. I expected Ned's personality to be as grotesque as his appearance. In a couple of days, I relaxed enough with him to discover that he was an earnest and endearing kid. His demeanor belied the hopelessness of his disease. Scared yes, ashamed yes, but he wanted to make contact, and he was intelligent and wise.

Ned is all that Dr. Ways really remembers about that clerkship. He dealt with other very sick children and learned about several rare pediatric problems but always under a shroud of fear, sadness, and anxiety evoked by Ned and sustained by other patients. Dr. Ways learned facts and concepts. What he didn't learn was how to deal with the "writhing mass" (his words) of powerful and frightening emotions, none of which he ever expressed to a colleague, an attending, or a resident. He had no warning of how emotionally wrenching this clerkship would be. Over the years, Dr. Ways learned that a lot of pediatrics is fun and gratifying. However, on that clerkship, he hated pediatrics and seriously questioned becoming a physician because of his powerful emotional reactions.

This story graphically portrays the impact of the implicit curriculum. Many clerkship experiences can be repugnant, sad, or painful. They can stimulate difficult memories and feelings, resurface unresolved personal issues, remind you of a loved one now dead, or all of the above. These impacts may be conscious or unconscious. *Of all aspects of clerkship education, students least expect the magnitude of its psychological and spiritual impact.* We see students initially open and outgoing toward their patients become self-absorbed, isolated, or depressed during a difficult clerkship. In contrast, on the rare clerkships where they receive appropriate support and attention, students can become more self-assured and open. We hope the self-care measures in Parts III and IV can help counteract any deleterious effects of your experience.

Environmental Aspects of the Implicit Curriculum

The Communication Environment

On most clerkships, there is a lot going on. Rounds can be disturbingly hectic. Pagers and telephones go off; people come and go. Some talk on their cell phone while standing or sitting among folks on rounds. Others read articles. Nearby conversations may make it difficult to hear the attending. Emergencies, such as codes, demand the presence of all or some of the house staff, and they can occur during rounds. Sometimes several emergencies occur at once.

Interruptions are often annoying. Third parties interrupt ongoing conversations with appalling regularity. The team is at the bedside when a consultant enters the room and speaks to the attending or resident. You are in the lounge with your resident reviewing a patient appraisal when another physician appears and without an, "excuse me," or an anticipatory pause will begin talking to your resident. In an emergency, this is understandable; otherwise it is rude. Interrupters seem to forget that everyone's busy; their anxiety about finishing one thing and getting on to the next pushes them to interrupt solely for their own convenience.

In an outpatient setting, the clerkship environment may be calmer. However, other members of the health care team are often hard to contact, or (because of demands elsewhere), they don't find as much time to spend with you as you would like.

Sights, Sounds, and Smells of the Environment

Visual vignettes are often powerful, moving, and emotionally difficult: a moribund patient lying passively, beyond hope, and with limited ability to communicate; people in profound suffering who cannot be helped by procedures or medications; gory injuries, deformities, decadence, and personal ruin. The patient in severe pain can be very difficult. Perhaps he or she has received all the pain medication that has been ordered. You want to do something but aren't sure what's best. These are difficult experiences even for seasoned physicians. Many doctors close themselves off from contact with such patients, usually unconsciously. *In this way, the physician shuts off meaningful communication between himself or herself and the patient who needs it the most.*

Smells may be troubling. The odors of disinfectants, urine, feces, and vomitus, are ineffectually countered by the more pleasant (but less frequent) smells of rubbing alcohol, scented soap, and clean sheets.

Finally, be ready for difficult sounds in the environment. Even in this era of the semiprivate room, repetitive moans, cries of pain, snoring, and babbles of confusion, fantasy, and hallucination are frequently heard. Unlike difficult sights, sounds may follow you anywhere; at times, they are impossible to escape. Mechanical and electronic tones add to the cacophony. Pagers (better now with vibrating ones), telephones, monitors, and the clatter that accompanies a code all play their own part in the "symphony of the service."

Sounds may have a profound effect on other patients. Repeated cries of pain and suffering, like water sluicing from a breached dam, can invade every corridor and every room. They awaken people and dishearten them. They can evoke great sympathy and a desire to help, but when felt as an outrageous invasion of peace and privacy, they can also stir up anger and impatience. One resident confessed the desire to scream "SHUT UP" but instead placated, comforted, or pleaded, knowing full well that the patient's moan was the only coping behavior left to him. We tend to "snow" such people with sedatives or analgesics. This is sometimes a reasonable course, but the choice should be individualized and is sometimes unwise. Further medication can exacerbate noisy behavior or provoke a dramatic dive into disorientation and hallucinations.

Some "Requirements" of the Implicit (Unstated) Curriculum

The implicit or hidden curriculum is driven by unspoken social and work expectations. Most attendings (attending physicians) and house staff anticipate these behaviors even when they do not mention them. Several of those listed below may be "expected" in any given clerkship. *When manifested consistently or in the extreme, they are definitely not all desirable or healthy—particularly 1, 2, and 3.*

1. Deal alone with psychologically difficult circumstances—repulsive, antagonistic, or dying patients, a failed code, suffering, pain, abuse. Be matter of fact or level-headed about such things. Work through fear, anxiety, and sorrow in private.

2. Be imperturbable. Act like a "mature male doctor" even though you're not yet a doctor and may not be a male. Do not show distress, anxiety, or fear when you deal with an emergency or other stress-provoking situation or show strong subjective reactions to a patient's sadness, mutilation, or suffering. Displaying frustration with the lab, X-ray people, or another department is usually OK.

3. If you must talk about your emotional reactions, don't approach attendings and most senior house staff; they won't have time anyway. Talk with student colleagues and "safe" house staff. Many will minimize your concerns or give facile reassurance instead of just hearing you out.

> The "bottom line" for 1, 2, and 3 is that you are supposed to act with "maturity" before you have sufficient experience to be mature.

4. Be supportive of and relatively unquestioning about all attempts to save life when the situation appears hopeless.

5. Be tolerant of attendings who talk too much, expect too much from you too soon, and are otherwise more of a hindrance than a help. The following whimsical anecdote illustrates this:

The professor of anatomy finished his orientation on surface anatomy to a group of first-year students. They were about to reenter the anatomy lab to begin Week 4. His concluding words were, "Now I expect you all to act like doctors." "But Dr. Kelly," said a student, "What do you mean, we've only been here three weeks." "Never mind, Thompson," Kelly replied, "You know exactly what I mean."

6. Observe "rights" of the house staff: to do certain procedures, to present your patient findings to the attending (most house staff are very fair about

this), to first interview a new patient when the service is busy. Also see Chapter 4 about supporting house staff.

In clerkships, in the anatomy lab, and in other settings, some of the major rules of the implicit curriculum govern the outward display of emotions. This is a two-edged sword. Some emotional damping helps you come to terms with the disturbing aspects of your experience. But when outward displays are controlled or throttled, inward reactions of anxiety, depression, fear, bad dreams, and sometimes severe disorders such as Post-Traumatic Stress Disorder occur. To escape, salve, or anesthetize psychic pain and turmoil, you may become cynical, indifferent, and further detach emotionally. While less common, students may abuse alcohol, other drugs, and food (see Chapters 17, 19).

To forestall negative outcomes, this book will pay close attention to the hidden curriculum as well as to the explicit one. We will offer many suggestions for healthy self-care (Chapters 15-19). We hope to help you create a healthier and more conscious overall clerkship experience.

3 Your Faculty I

Attending Physicians

You are a student doctor and a lot like a rookie in the major leagues. The attending physicians are your manager and coaches, and the house staff members are veteran players with significantly more experience. This chapter will prepare you to work with attending physicians. (House staff and others are discussed in the next chapter.) We will emphasize windows of opportunity and alert you to possible shortcomings.

Profile of the Attending Physician

The attending is the chief doctor on your assigned unit with ultimate responsibility for quality patient care. Your attending physician may be a full- or part-time faculty member or a physician in private practice with a "clinical faculty" appointment. Residents and students report to and seek advice from him or her about difficult medical or administrative problems. The attending also has leadership responsibility for education on the service. He or she makes rounds (Chapter 10) daily or every other day but will not necessarily see or discuss every patient every time. Although with the student(s) only a few hours a week, the attending has a lot to say about student evaluation.

The attitudes, values, interpersonal style, and teaching style of attendings vary. A few exhibit remarkable sensitivity to patients; some are devoted to teaching and do it well. Others talk in monotones, discuss only technical diagnostic and management issues, and may appear uncomfortable in their physician or teaching role. Like college and many graduate school faculty members,

DEFINITIONS

Attending physician: The physician with ultimate responsibility for patients. The attending serves for two to eight weeks at a time, conducts rounds with house staff and/or students, and is generally available for advice 24 hours a day. In some hospitals, patients may have different attendings, each responsible for their own patients.

Preceptor: A faculty member, advanced resident, or fellow who teaches students, but in this time period does not conduct rounds with house staff and is not responsible for patient care on the service. He or she meets with students three to five times a week for one to two hours when students present and discuss patients. A preceptor also reads and criticizes student write-ups and progress notes.

Clerkship coordinator: An attending physician and/or faculty person who organizes, administrates, and monitors the clerkship experience for one specialty at a particular hospital or clinic.

Mentor: Usually a faculty member who may or may not also be (at some time) your attending. A mentor invests time and concern in you by serving as a guide and counselor on career and professional matters and sometimes personal ones as well.

House staff: A collective term for residents (PGY-1, PGY-2, PGY-3)[a] in training. House staff assigned to the service will help you learn techniques such as venepuncture, arterial sticks, thoracentesis, and abdominal and spinal taps. They may read and critique your progress notes and "work-ups." *Intern* is the same as a PGY-1. The term is still used in some places.

Fellow: Most *fellows* have finished a residency in and are now being trained in a subspecialty such as cardiology or gastroenterology. They do a combination of research, teaching, and patient care.

Full-time faculty: Faculty members paid a full-time salary by the medical school for their services in patient care, administration, research, and teaching.

Part-time faculty: Also have a part-time private or HMO practice. They may be paid for time spent in medical school activities.

Private practitioner: Physicians who are in the private or HMO practice of medicine. They may be part-time faculty and are probably not paid for teaching.

---

a. Postgraduate years 1, 2, and 3.

medical teachers are better and more focused on *teaching at* (shoveling information at students) than *facilitating learning* (helping students acquire "the art of the utilization of knowledge," Whitehead, 1957), which includes processes such as interviewing and effective, useful problem solving. Too many bring a reductionistic perspective to their instruction; they teach disease-oriented details before ascertaining your grasp of the broader picture. Although unfortunate, such limitations are understandable. The confidence and expertise of attendings is in their area of specialization. Full-time faculty are hired, promoted, acclaimed, and financially rewarded primarily on the basis of their credentials as researcher, specialist, or subspecialist. On rounds, they tend to expound about and ask questions in these areas.

Staffing Patterns

The most common inpatient clerkship staffing pattern comprises an attending physician, one or more residents, and one or more medical students. Most often, the attending teaches students and house staff together, but on some clerkships, he or she will preceptor students separately. Rarely, there will be a second faculty preceptor who is responsible only for the students. If assigned to such a preceptor (a seriously endangered species), your group will meet him or her two to three times a week. The time may be devoted to rounds on your patients, informal discussion, and topic presentations. Most preceptors are good generalists and can help you with problem-solving and physical examination skills.

You may be assigned to a community hospital clerkship where there are no house staff. Also, you may have different attendings for different patients.

Activity: Imagine yourself in the role of attending physician for a day. How does it feel? What do you do well? What are problems for you? Why?

The Good Teachers

The better teachers will impress you with their knowledge of the material, and/or certain of their qualities and professional behaviors will appeal to you. You may find yourself imitating them. In judging these factors, try to distinguish between pedantic show-off stuff and real depth of useful knowledge and skills.

The effective teacher will inspire you to learn bountifully from each of your patients but is not always charismatic. One of our most effective teachers in medical school seemed boring, but he taught an invaluable, disciplined approach to the medical history that has stood the test of time (see Chapter 5).

Emulate the instructor who keeps rounds moving and is well organized. He or she teaches you to define and resolve problems by requiring (a) clear problem statements derived from an adequate database, (b) prioritization of those problems with respect to clinical urgency and overall patient well-being, (c) plans for solving the most urgent problems, (d) the establishment of management goals, and (e) suggestions for monitoring progress (Chapter 5). Don't judge your teachers solely on the number of facts and concepts they dispense. The qualities of leadership; orderly problem solving; good judgment; the ability to say, "I don't know, but we can look it up"; kindness; respect; and empathy are also important.

You can learn from attendings by watching them at work, not just by listening to their fund of knowledge or asking them questions. Dr. Janes's focused attention saved an intern's life:

> Rigley was a 26-year-old intern. While attending a film, he developed a severe headache and sore neck. Two hours later, he dropped a dish and said his walking felt awkward. In the ER, his temperature was 103, his neck was stiff, and he had bilateral Babinski reflexes. He quickly slipped into coma. The resident removed cerebrospinal fluid (CSF). CSF protein was normal, the sugar borderline, and only a few cells were seen. Gram's stain was also negative. The resident plated the CSF for culture. Twelve hours later no growth was visible, but the attending, Dr. Janes, swabbed the surface of the plate and stained it anyway. The Gram's stain revealed bacteria typical for meningococcal meningitis. Appropriate treatment was begun. Within 24 hours, Rigley was conscious and a week later virtually well with no residua.

Look for attendings who set a good example—who behave with house staff, students, and other staff, in a kind, respectful, and nourishing manner. Pay special attention to the teacher who surprises or pleases you with his or her behavior toward patients. Some are extraordinarily gifted in their manner and sensitivity toward patients and in the ease with which they relate to them.

Don't forget: Observing your faculty in action will help you determine what values and behaviors you want to manifest (or not have) as a physician.

Shortcomings

Like all of us, attending physicians have shortcomings. In general, they fall into four categories: deficient teaching skills, difficult personality characteristics, discomfort with charged emotional issues (such as addiction, deterioration, disfigurement, dying, and other forms of suffering), and poor expression and clarification of values.

Teaching Skill

Undeniably, some who teach clinical medicine are good, a few even wonderful, teachers. However, many are not, and some may be of little or no value as instructors. Despite this, it's best to assume that all have something to offer.

A lot has been learned in the last two decades about helping clinicians become better teachers, but it is far from universally applied. Even full-time academic physicians are not held accountable on their ability to teach, guide, and model behavior. Apparently, it is assumed that, as physicians, they are miraculously qualified to teach others. For practitioners far distant from an academic teaching center, such laxity is often not germane; applied to those who teach regularly, it is educational malpractice.

Personality Traits

A knowledgeable attending may have an abrasive, overbearing (occasionally unbearable!) personality and/or excessive need for control. He or she may be harsh or discounting with patients and students. In such circumstances, the best approach is to behave respectfully yourself. Heed Osler's (1932a, p. 3) plea for imperturbability. **Treat your patients and teachers with caring and respect, no matter how a teacher may affect you.** Your behavior may catalyze someone else to change; you become a good influence without sticking your neck out.

Although the situation has improved, we still observe sexist and racist behaviors among attendings. Harassment occurs. On recently completing her surgery clerkship, a female student was told by an attending that because she was married and had two children, she shouldn't consider surgery. This story is all too common. Women experience subtle and overt sexism, harassment, and discrimination and (as faculty) are promoted less often (Coombs, 1998). Add usually greater home and family responsibilities and a woman's passage through medical school (and service as faculty) is significantly more difficult than her male colleague's.

Discomfort With Emotional and Spiritual Issues

Faculty performance is often hindered by inadequate emotional sensitivity and counseling skills. It is difficult for some attendings to engage with patients and trainees in a full and genuine way. The emotional challenges of medical school are many. Patients' psychological issues are vitally important. Ignoring the need for most teachers to be sensitized and trained to model, interact, and teach in the affective realms is a serious shortcoming of medical education.

Values Clarification

At times, you will question certain aspects of patient care—for example, choice of treatment or the continuation of extreme measures when all hope of quality life appears lost. When you disagree, it is important, as a concerned caregiver, to speak up at an appropriate time. Unfortunately, in our experience, many faculty do not seize upon such opportunities to engage in mutual values clarification with the student(s). So, be circumspect. If there is potentially serious conflict with a faculty member, seek out a mediator or ombudsman.

* * *

By and large, attending physicians are valuable, hardworking, well-meaning individuals. Some are exceedingly good teachers, and many work hard to overcome their shortcomings. Unfortunately, many physicians' teaching and counseling skills and their sensitivities about the emotional and spiritual issues of their patients and trainees do not improve with time. Habits learned in training are hard to break.

The teacher-student relationship is complex. More of its intricacies are discussed in Chapters 8 (Communication) and 10 (Rounds and Teamwork).

4 Faculty II

House Staff, Nurses, and Others

On clerkships, smart, friendly students add another arm to the workforce and bring welcome variety and humor. But when nurses, residents, or other staff members orient you or demonstrate a technique, they are repeating tasks they do with most new medical students. As Gusky (1982, p. 27) points out, you are extra work for them. You are on their turf, not yours. By acknowledging these points, you will get a lot of help and attention.

Activity: During your first days on service, observe closely and spend time with the residents, the charge nurse, an orderly, and the unit secretary. Ask each about his or her main job. How does it relate to the work of others? Does it involve interaction with medical students? What is difficult about having medical students here? What has been your best experience with medical students? What advice do you have for me? This will be time well spent.

House Staff

Interns and residents will be your most important teachers. Many like to teach, some do it a lot, and a few are very good. These teaching sessions will vary in frequency and length of contact (a half-minute to a half-hour) and be mostly informal—at the bedside or sitting around the chart rack.

Teaching Patterns and Style of House Staff

Typically, house staff teach in bytes that capitalize on opportunities and "teachable moments." Interns teach as things happen or procedures need doing. The old adage "see one, do one, teach one" is still faithful to reality. The success of each learning moment depends on the participants' level of fatigue and other responsibilities.

There will be brief transfers of information or suggestions such as, "You should examine Mr. Smith's abdomen." These moments are spontaneous, pragmatic, and occur frequently on work and attending rounds. Jot down the suggestions in your notebook because you may be doing something else when the suggestion comes. From interns, you may get brief comments on your write-ups but rarely a whole review.

Advanced residents (PGY-2 or PGY-3) may go over some of your workups in detail and suggest improvements in your histories and physical exams (PEs). They are good at this—because experience is an exceptional teacher when it comes to the interview history and PE. **If your write-ups are not being reviewed by residents or attendings, tell them. This is something you value and need.**

Advanced residents and fellows are more confident, usually less rushed, and a little more formal. They may schedule special teaching conferences for your student group that may not be at the best times for you. Go anyway if possible. Busy residents appreciate your attendance. You will learn most in sessions keyed to a patient to whom you are assigned.

House staff or subspecialty fellows will help you learn new techniques, such as arterial puncture, spinal tap, taking EKGs, nasogastric intubation, and doing blood cultures. Although they expect a lot of you in terms of chores (scut work), house staff members are, for the most part, your allies and colleagues during a clerkship.

Special Case of the Intern or PGY-1

Interns have a demanding job. In July and August, they are fresh out of medical school, so many will be in new surroundings where rules and procedures may be unfamiliar to them. The attending staff and more advanced residents are strangers to them. They are often lonely. The workload may be more diffi-

cult and frustrating than they expected, and they may be constantly sleep deprived. Early in the internship year, you, as a student, may know more about the
service than they do, and you can be particularly helpful to them.

On most inpatient services, your work will closely approximate that of the
interns with fewer assigned patients. If they're good, they will model what is
expected of you. Don't take their haste and (sometimes) irritability personally.
Some days, they may be alarmingly tired and grouchy.

We have paraphrased the following "intern priorities" (Lederman, 1995,
p. 11). **Help the intern meet them and you will get more of his or her time.**

1. Complete the daily care of ongoing patients as soon as possible.

2. Promptly appraise (Chapter 9) and propose management for each new
   patient assigned to you.

3. Help discharge or transfer suitable patients.

4. Minimize distractions and unimportant phone calls from nurses and others.

5. Ensure a smooth flow of ward activities.

6. SLEEP.

The priorities of senior house staff are usually the same as the intern's. Draw
the "bloods," put the lab results in the chart, complete the history and PE and
record it in the chart, talk to the family, do procedures, schedule consultations,
make sure orders are written and countersigned. These are all subsets of intern
Priorities 1 and 2 above.

While it's not recommended that you openly address house staff by the nicknames ("operational role") in Table 4.1, it will be fun for you and your colleagues to see who fits in what category.

Teaching Skills of House Staff

Only a few residency programs devote time to train house staff as teachers.
There are some things you can do to improve teaching on your clerkships.

Activity: To improve house staff teaching:
- Aid the intern priorities given above.
- Do your patient appraisals (H&Ps) and ward chores promptly.

Table 4.1 Humorous Classification of Resident Types

Nickname	Operational Role	Typical Behavior
Gunner	Mr. Please Everyone, Do Everything	Shoots from the hip; aims to please; gung ho
Rip Van Winkle	Sleepwalker	Falls asleep writing, at conferences, and sometimes even standing up!
Nerd	Dr. Precise; by-the-book (his or her book)	Pedantic, bossy; quotes literature all the time
Real Doctor	One of us	Competent, considerate, honors patients, listens, teaches responsibly
Lame Duck	Out of here	Has only a few days left on this assignment and is living in the future
Dr. Mystery	Masked woman or man	Hard to read; motives not clear; may work well but closed about self

- Negotiate extra teaching for extra work.
- If you read new material related to a topic one of the residents discussed with you, share your learning with the resident.
- When they briefly discuss a particular topic, ask pertinent questions.
- After a teaching-learning exchange, summarize what you've learned and ask for feedback.

Cautionary Advice

Remembering their own medical school years, most residents are basically kind and respectful to medical students. However, be alert for the following resident behaviors and counter them if possible.

- An occasional intern will try to adopt you as his or her private scut person and ward "managerette." He or she may expect far more scut work than you can profit from—or even complete.
- Sometimes, particularly early in the third year, it can feel like you've been given more responsibility than you want (see Chapter 5).

- House staff, like attendings, emphasize facts and concepts. They are more comfortable discussing pathophysiology, pills, and procedures than a patient's psychological issues and poverty of spirit. *Because in most cases, it is essential to discuss the cognitive material, it won't always be easy for you to bring up neglected emotional and spiritual issues.* Do your best!

- The following behaviors are clues that a resident is skirting the patient's affective concerns or stumbling over his or her own hang-ups:
  - Failing to ask an obviously suffering patient about his or her pain or emotional state
  - Using jokes as the major way of relating to the same patient
  - Not acknowledging and discussing expressions (even subtle ones) of anger or frustration from a patient
  - A repetitively "cheerful mouth" or facile approach to a patient; unjustified rather than genuine reassurance

The Nursing Staff

Talented professionals in their own right, nurses can be a great source of wisdom and aid. Early in the clerkship, observe carefully what goes on and who does what (see activity at the beginning of this chapter). Learn how the nurses are organized to do their work. Some places assign each nurse to a few patients for whom he or she does everything. Other units divide the tasks: One nurse delivers the medications to every patient on the service, another does special treatments, and so on. **Make sure they know that you know how they work.** This is an essential principle of respect, and it facilitates good patient care.

The nursing staff can supplement your learning. Many have a great fund of valuable knowledge. For example, on surgery, the nurses will know about postop care: electrolyte and fluid replacement, when patients should be ambulated, and/or catheterized, and monitoring urine flow. Nurses can teach you certain essential aspects of patient care that are seldom taught by physician faculty: turning patients to avoid bedsores; placement of IV lines, central venous catheters, various nasogastric and other tubes; management and operation of respirators; and the setup and use of monitors. On critical care units, they can teach you to monitor patients, help you do CPR if necessary, and assist with other aspects of life support.

Some will be good teachers and some will not. **Pay attention, be respectful, and listen. You will gain their support.** Undisputedly, the respect of the nursing staff can significantly increase the value of your clerkship experience—sometimes magically.

Nurses are valuable to you for other reasons (Gusky, 1982, pp. 45-47):

- They will warn you if you get in over your head, and/or are about to commit a mistake (particularly if they see you as an ally).
- Working with the better attendings, they know how to resolve certain difficulties in patient care.
- When you are away from the unit, they can inform you about ongoing or incipient problems, and they may perform work that you forgot to do—saving you significant embarrassment.

If they see you as an ally, your relationship with nurses can be the difference between a great clerkship and a mediocre one. **The cardinal rule is do not speak or act "down" to nurses.** They are acutely sensitized to arrogance and condescension and will blacklist you early if they think you feel superior or regard them as less competent.

Sometimes, your relationship with nursing staff can be tricky. "Some nursing supervisors specify . . . no fraternizing" (Coombs, 1998, p. 109) and that formal address be used. In many settings, however, a first-name basis is customary. Unfortunately, a few nurses seem compelled to make a student's or resident's life difficult, just as a few residents and attendings can make a nurse's life difficult. Subtle sabotage, triangulation, and an inappropriate need for control is not unknown. To avoid these eventualities, keep a low profile early in your stay on a service, make a point of asking for help in understanding how the service works, listen carefully, and follow their advice. The most difficult of nurses usually respond to kindness and respect.

Other Professionals and Paraprofessionals as Instructors

Unit Secretary or Clerk

This individual deserves special mention. Administratively, he or she is usually in the nursing department. The responsibilities of clerks vary, but they usually function as the chief communication officer. They keep charts available and up to date, schedule X-rays and other special procedures, know where patients are, make up the new (blank) chart for newly admitted patients, and relay treatment orders to central supply, pharmacy, and other special services. They are like air traffic controllers in commercial aviation. An effective clerk makes all the difference in the functioning of a ward, unit, or service. **You must spend time with the unit secretary at the beginning of your clerkship so as to understand their responsibilities and how to cooperate with them.**

Nurse Practitioners, Physician Assistants, Paramedics

At some point, you will work with nurse practitioners (NPs) and physician's assistants (PAs). The more you learn about their training and expertise (widely variable), the better. Many of them do a lot of teaching. Their approach is usually quite practical. True humility is of the essence here. You can learn from practitioners at any level, and you'll find nurse clinicians, PAs, or paramedics of enormous value to you.

A student took an elective in cardiac rehabilitation. Joe D, a paramedic experienced in critical care, was assigned to the exercise sessions. Every two or three weeks, one patient or another experienced chest pain, dizziness, or exceptional shortness of breath, and there was one episode of cardiac arrest. In each instance, the student worked side by side with the paramedic to decide what was going on and what needed to be done. Years later, the student regarded that association as the time he learned most about evaluating a high-risk patient with new symptoms.

Other Professional Caregivers

In the course of clerkships, you will encounter pharmacists, social workers, nutritionists, physical and occupational therapists, lab personnel (med techs), hospice workers, and other caregivers. Some will be on the everyday patient care team. Others will be consultants. You may learn most from them through their notes in the chart.

Most of these people will have a lot to offer. Although you are still a student, many will defer to you. Encourage them to state their opinion; it will be worth hearing. Your responsibilities will make it impossible to speak directly to everyone who sees your patients. However, do it when possible, particularly if you have requested the consult.

Chapter 10 on rounds will discuss further aspects of your relationships with teachers, consultants, and other staff members.

5 The Discipline of Patient Care

We regard discipline as a consistent set of behaviors, based on personal choices, that furthers our lives in a useful and usually gratifying way. It may be modeled by a parent or mentor. Commonly, the rewards are not immediately apparent. The word *discipline* comes from the Latin *discipolus*, which freely translates to "learn."

As a third-year clerk on internal medicine, Ways and 10 other students met weekly with a venerable professor for $2\frac{1}{2}$ hours to review one student's history and physical exam. Dr. Atchley was kind, forceful, and detailed in his approach, and although he engaged everyone, the class often felt totally bored. But after 12 sessions, they were all very advanced in the skills of history taking and had a deep appreciation of why an expert medical history includes so many items— some of which seemed superfluous to us until they had been "Atchleyized." For example, Ways presented a 48-year-old man with congestive heart failure, cardiac enlargement, and a heart murmur. "Ways," said Dr. Atchley, "I notice that your list of childhood diseases does not mention scarlet fever." Ways acknowledged that he hadn't asked about scarlet fever. "Why might that be important in this case?" Ways wasn't sure, but one of the "gunners" in the group offered that scarlet fever was caused by beta-hemolytic strep, and it could be followed by rheumatic fever. Acute rheumatic fever was then the most common cause of valvular heart disease. When questioned, the patient recalled a prolonged illness at the age of eight with intermittent fever and some joint pain; he might well have had

31

low-grade rheumatic fever. After further studies, the patient's basic heart problem turned out to be stenosis of the mitral valve, one classic manifestation of rheumatic heart disease.

For years, fellow house staff, attending physicians, and chiefs of service praised Ways's patient appraisals. He and his classmates were a step ahead of house staff trained in other schools in their ability to elicit and record a patient history that was a profound diagnostic tool and a facilitator of good management. Some fellow residents clearly knew more facts than Ways, but their mastery of the diagnostic process was not as accomplished.

In addition to honoring the patient (Chapter 7), the elements of discipline essential to quality doctoring are responsibility, honesty, delayed gratification, and balancing. These are qualities that you willingly choose or neglect. They are the essence of maturity and of being a good physician.

Responsibility

There are three important aspects of responsibility related to your clerkships.

First, it's up to you to have the best experience possible. Not all clerkships are of the same quality. But if you accept responsibility for your part in making each of them successful and focus on the positive aspects, all of them will be profitable. In our clerkship study, some students repeatedly made negative remarks early in their rotation. As a consequence, their lenses were wrinkled and their view of what happened, altered. Be on guard for negativity, especially when you are tired, sleep deprived, and frustrated.

Second, get a clear picture of what is expected of you and how you can be a valued member of the team (see Box 5.1). Then be diligent in getting the job done. This requires checking repeatedly about what is expected and requesting feedback at appropriate intervals.

Third, don't be a victim. Your attending may be chronically late, superficial, and inattentive. You may be assigned "too many" cardiac patients or old people. Your intern may hog procedures. These are all regrettable but, despite them, make the clerkship a positive experience. Counter them with energy and creativity. Read up on and interview patients other than your own. Arrange and attend family meetings. Organize informal teaching conferences with subspecialty consultants.

Joe and Edith, two third-year students, were assigned to a community hospital clerkship in internal medicine. It was the first clerkship ever

---

BOX 5.1

The Valued Clinical Clerk

- Stays up to date on patients; chases down lab work, X-rays
- Finishes workups promptly, gets write-ups into charts
- Accepts new patients without fussing about "another this or that"
- Hangs around for night on-call, even when it's quiet
- Reads up on patient's problems
- Tailors presentations to the needs of particular rounds and to the load of that day
- Is routinely thorough before being brilliantly focused (this can change as you gain experience)
- Does most of what he or she needs to do without being asked, certainly not twice
- Appears neat
- Anticipates needs at bedside during/before rounds
- Responds to questions honestly with "I don't know" when he or she doesn't, plus "I will find out and report back to you"
- Has obvious rapport with patients, speaks to them at bedside, introduces other people to patient—explains who they are
- Finds out to whom, how, and what to communicate with nursing staff

---

held in that hospital. The attendings had limited teaching experience, and there was no house staff. Joe complained to friends and his adviser that this was an inferior experience. He did his work but didn't go past the minimal requirements and was "out of there" at 5:00 p.m. except when on-call. Edith, by contrast, quickly became famous for her perceptive and useful questions, which spared no one. She was relaxed with her patients and unearthed important issues—some missed by the physicians. She did her "scut" promptly without complaint. She systematically studied the extent to which important lab results were "missed" by the physicians and devised a way to flag abnormal results. Two years later, in residency, the chief of service told

her that her dean's letter included detailed quotes from her evaluation on that clerkship. They had strongly influenced him to rank her
highly in the matching plan.

How do you, as a student, decide how much responsibility to assume in the
care of your patients? One day, the nurse informs you that Mr. Edwards's intravenous fluid orders have run out. The intern is unavailable; the resident is leading a conference in another part of the hospital. Do you write an order to add
another bag of electrolytes or not?

Or your patient, a 55-year-old man, is scheduled for a barium enema. Thirty
minutes before it is to begin, he feels nauseated and complains of vague pre-
cordial pain. The hospital has no house staff, and the patient's own doctor left
town last night for a professional meeting. The physician to whom he signed
out has not yet seen this patient and is unavailable for the next 10 to 15 minutes.
Do you cancel the barium study, ask for a stat cardiology consult, run an EKG
yourself and send some enzyme studies to the lab, or do all (or none) of the
above? Dilemmas such as these occur.

Often, it is difficult to know how much responsibility to take. In a life-threatening situation, if you are the only physician or medical student available, team
up with the nearest nurse and do what needs to be done—to the best of your
combined knowledge. If the situation does not appear immediately life threatening, err on the side of taking too little responsibility. Both of the patients
sketched above can wait a few more minutes while you try to find expert help,
although the second patient is more vulnerable than the first and should be directly observed until he is on a monitor. If you're working in a hospital (especially one that has an ER), there will be someone not far away who can help and
advise you. When you start your clerkship, it is your responsibility to find out
where you can turn under such circumstances.

**The bottom line: Don't take on more than you are a little uncomfortable
with. Beware of cockiness, a subterfuge of the ego.**

Activity: Table 5.1 describes several situations you may encounter.
There are blank spaces for you to add others that threaten you. Using the
scale at the bottom of the table, register your degree of discomfort with
each of them in the "first week" of the clerkship. Discuss your responses
with an attending or a resident. After four weeks and at the end of the
clerkship, rate each of the circumstances again.

Table 5.1   Discomfort Assessment

Conditions	Week 1	Week 4	End
Cardiopulmonary resuscitation			
Telling family members that their loved one has rapidly fatal cancer			
Doing your first arterial stick after only reviewing an instructional video			
Talking to a patient about their sexual habits and experience			
Examining your first patient with AIDS and a vigorous productive cough			
Evaluating a patient with severe shortness of breath before the PGY-1[a] sees her			
Telling a mother that her six-month old baby boy has a heart murmur			
Continuing with an interview when a patient is openly hostile			
Student to add			
Student to add			
Student to add			

a. PGY-1 refers to the first postgraduate year.
Discomfort index: 0 = No conscious awareness of discomfort
                1 = Mind does not admit discomfort, but heart pounds or stomach feels
                     queasy or sweating is noticeable: i.e., bodily changes suggest discomfort
                2 = Definitely uncomfortable in body or mind
                3 = So uncomfortable that you would rather not do this

Honesty

Four aspects of honesty are particularly germane to clinical work:

1. Accurate reporting of data

2. Being truthful about what you don't know

3. Knowing when and where to speak out your opinions and judgments

4. Acknowledging errors in clinical judgment and decision making

The first three are straightforward. The fourth is more complex. See also honesty in Chapter 7.

Accurate Reporting of Data

The medical student assigned to a new patient usually elicits and reports the most comprehensive history and physical exam. Your write-up is used in diagnosis and management and may become part of the official medical record. As you write, you realize that you neglected certain questions or omitted something in the physical exam. It is essential to *either* return to the patient immediately and get the data (simply say, "I forgot to . . ."; patients understand) *or* write "not elicited" or "not done" in the write-up. **Don't report something as "negative" or "normal" when you haven't asked the question or done the exam.** Omissions are commonplace and understandable. Falsification is a doorway to trouble.

Acknowledging That You Don't Know

When asked a question that they don't know how to answer, some students will hem and haw; others will guess. It is refreshing and far more disciplined to hear a straightforward "I don't know." Teachers will be more impressed by a clerk who is honest in this way than by one who guesses or suggests faintly plausible answers.

Voicing Judgments and Opinions

If your clinical judgment differs from the house staff's or attending's, it is important to offer it. Someone will learn. When to offer it is a separate decision. In an emergency, speak up immediately if your opinion might alter the course of treatment. In nonemergencies, offering an alternative diagnosis or treatment is usually best done away from the patient so it can be discussed.

Treat opinions or judgments about colleagues and teachers carefully. For example, if you think your attending is condescending, it serves no one well, least of all yourself, to make that opinion known. However, if he or she consistently treats patients abrasively or with indifference, consult with house staff or another attending physician. The offending physician may have a mental health or addiction problem that is threatening his or her life and work.

Acknowledging Errors in Judgment/Decision Making

First, acknowledge the extent to which you are responsible when something doesn't go as planned or is forgotten (e.g., needed data is not available for rounds).

A medical student, Francoise, admitted a 52-year-old man after 24 hours of severe upper abdominal pain and vomiting. The patient had been drinking heavily for several weeks. Blood chemistries, including a serum amylase (a test to detect acute pancreatitis), were ordered. The upper-GI series suggested a gastric ulcer, so intravenous fluids, antacids, and drug therapy to inhibit gastric secretions were begun. The morning after admission, the patient's lab sheet showed a normal serum amylase. It was in the wrong chart, but Francoise did not check the name on the slip. On rounds, she reported the value as normal. The patient was not improving. His pain and vomiting continued, and his blood pressure and serum calcium were low. Puzzled, the attending and residents leafed through the lab work and discovered that the amylase report was for another patient. A call to the lab revealed the correct amylase to be quite elevated—the patient had acute pancreatitis—a problem that can be fatal if not treated promptly. Fortunately, Mr. Stone recovered. The student acknowledged her error at the end of rounds without implicating the ward clerk who had posted the slip in the chart.

Second, know that *errors are frequent in medicine.* Carl Jung and many others have emphasized that individuation must include mistakes—growth requires them. Table 5.2 distinguishes different degrees of clinical errors and their consequences.

In her *Unity of Mistakes,* Tracy Paget (1988) agrees that errors are made frequently in medicine. She calls medicine an "error-ridden activity." She states further that "accounts by physicians . . . report that mistakes are inevitable—that is, that medical mistakes are an intrinsic feature of medical work." And later, she points out that the topic of mistakes in medicine, "is far broader than errors 'of negligence.' " (pp. 15, 133). Robert Hilfiker (1991) speaks ardently to the paradox: "I am a healer, yet I sometimes do more harm than good." He repeatedly points out that errors can have drastic consequences (although most do not), that there are abundant opportunities to make them (for all doctors), that they often leave us uncertain about our culpability, and that despite all this,

Table 5.2   Clinical Errors

Error identified in time:	Some errors are identified and corrected before adverse effects occur and THERE IS NO EFFECT ON PATIENT'S COURSE.
Gray zone:	Other errors are discovered in conjunction with demonstrable impact but are CORRECTED BEFORE NEGATIVELY AFFECTING PATIENT'S COURSE.
Definite mistake:	Still other errors are damaging; they are missed for some time or never detected. THERE IS DEFINITE OR POTENTIAL ADVERSE EFFECT ON PATIENT'S COURSE.

there is powerful denial among colleague physicians that mistakes do happen. This creates an "intolerable dilemma." "We see the horror of our mistakes, yet we cannot deal with their enormous emotional impact" (p. 386).

The most pervasive problem with mistakes in medicine is that they are concealed. People are afraid they'll lose their jobs, be held in contempt, be sued, or be otherwise devalued if they talk about their mistakes. We believe that the consequences of honesty are less punishing than the consequences of hiding them. There is deep sorrow for the provider embedded in his or her error, and this needs to be processed with other people. If mistakes are kept secret, this does not happen.

We must minimize mistakes with untiring vigilance: We must find ways to deal forthrightly with those that do occur. Failing in this, both as individuals and as a professional group, we resort to unhealthy ways to contain our pain. Hilfiker (1991) notes:

> Little wonder, that physicians are accused of playing God. Little wonder that we are defensive about our judgments, that we blame the patient or the previous physician when things go wrong, that we yell at nurses for their mistakes, that we have such high rates of alcoholism, drug addiction, and suicide.
>
> At some point, we must all bring medical mistakes out of the closet. This will be difficult as long as both the profession and society continue to project their desires for perfection onto the doctor. Physicians need permission to admit errors. They need permission to share them with their patients. The practice of medicine is difficult enough without having to bear the yoke of perfection" (pp. 386-387).

If you (or a colleague) are making errors frequently, consider the possibility of sleep deprivation (see Chapter 13). Many students get less sleep than they need but are in denial about how significantly this can influence performance. Frequent mistakes or incomplete work can certainly be a symptom of those conditions. Some students will abuse alcohol or other drugs; very rarely, one will have an enlarging brain tumor or psychosis.

When involved in a mistake, be forthright like Francoise. Acknowledge whatever responsibility you may have.

Do you or don't you tell a patient about a mistake. This can be tricky. If the error has had unfavorable impact, the patient may take you to court or you may lose that person as a patient. He or she may publicize your error making. While these are realistic possibilities, being forthright is the best course, and it is mandatory if the patient's clinical course and/or life are affected. Contrast the following stories:

Story 1: A healthy, athletic, 52-year-old man had sudden onset of abdominal pain. After a week of vomiting and fever, the diagnosis of Crohn's disease was made. He was treated for seven weeks on total parenteral feeding and IV antibiotics. Surgery at that time revealed no evidence of Crohn's disease; rather, 8 weeks before, he had perforated his appendix.

Story 2: Dr. K. ordered ankle X-rays for an injured athlete. The films showed a break in the distal fibula, but this did not correspond with the physical findings. The films had been cross-labeled with another set taken the same hour. Repeat X-rays of Dr. K's patient revealed no fracture. Dr. K elected not to tell the patient about the mislabeling.

Story 3: Dr. M was covering a vacationing colleague's practice. The first day she saw a 40-year-old woman with known metastatic cancer. A follow-up chest X-ray, ordered by the patient's regular doctor, showed a cancer nodule in the lung with metastatic nodes in the mediastinum. Previous chest films were reported normal. In reviewing these earlier films, the radiologist said abnormal findings, although less obvious, were present three months before.

In Story 1, it would have been unconscionable not to reveal the error to the patient. In Story 2, the physician chose to stay mum arguing that the error was discovered in time to correct it without consequences for the patient. Story 3 is

Table 5.3   Low-Gratification Tasks

Internal Medicine	Pediatrics	OB-GYN
Delivering specimens to the lab	Ear exam on crying infant	Pap smears
Rectal exam	Drawing blood on infant	Catheterization
Emptying bedpan	Gastric intubation of a toddler	Taking a history on Gravida VI, Para V woman

more ambiguous. Dr. M could wait and let the patient's regular doctor tell her about the earlier films, or Dr. M. could reveal the error herself. What would you do?

Delayed Gratification

Delayed gratification is the easiest discipline to understand, but for some, it's the hardest to follow! **It requires doing what needs to be done before doing what may be more fun and often easier.** Desserts come last.

As a clinical clerk, you do a number of things that are less fun than others or no fun at all but that are, nevertheless, a necessary part of the role. They vary from clerkship to clerkship. Table 5.3 is one student's list for internal medicine, surgery, and OB-GYN clerkships. They may or may not coincide with your choices.

If the mundane or unpleasant tasks are seen as a "drag" instead of as an important part of the job, they become even less gratifying. Finding reward in the ungratifying aspects of a job is a big secret of job satisfaction. Often, if you're fortunate, a low-gratification task becomes a pleasure and turns itself into an integrated high priority.

Balancing

Psychiatrist and philosopher, Scott Peck (1978) says *balancing is the "discipline required to discipline discipline"* [italics added] (p. 64).

Many students and physicians are also spouses and parents. They may also believe passionately in some cause. When their medical work consumes 50 to 60 hours a week, they are hard-pressed to balance their lives. Unexpected opportunities to enrich any of these roles (such as being a Little League coach or giving a professional paper) may complicate their lives further.

Discipline requires not only resolve but also flexibility. "Balancing is the discipline that gives us flexibility" (Peck, 1978, p. 64). In a sense, it is both the tachometer and the internal feedback loop, or cybernetic, of discipline.

Peck feels that the essence of balancing is "giving up" (p. 66). It is impossible to do most clerkships in a full way without sidetracking certain cherished aspects of your life. Hopefully, you will not give them up for good. If you are compelled to provide frequently for friends' needs, from one perspective certainly altruistic, you must give some of that up. Rejecting responsibility that is not fundamentally or healthfully ours is, itself, being responsible.

Because certain activities (reading, meditating, basketball, prayer, dancing—done perhaps even in a disciplined way) help you live the rest of your life more fully and competently, it is important to balance your work with some of those activities. **Although you must give up some things during the clerkship, be clear that you won't give up something essential to your well-being.** You may diminish the time you spend on it, but don't give it up.

Picture a balancing scale. Keep it balanced rather than always dipping to one side. In balance, it can seesaw, and perhaps rotate; out of balance, it's stuck. You will probably need to move the fulcrum during clerkships so there's less relaxation and fun, and more work, but you're OK as long as the work side doesn't hit the ground. That's painful, and you will be stuck. The balancing we must do is important to our patients as well.

Activity:

1. List 3-4 tasks that are low gratification for you.
2. List areas in your life where balancing is pertinent.
3. Note that balancing self-care (in its broadest meaning) and work is a central theme of this book.
4. What are some activities that can offset the work side of your scale?

In Chapters 15 and 16, there are self-care boxes. They will help you balance care of yourself against the emotional, spiritual, physical, and cognitive demands made by your work. Part IV is entirely devoted to self-care.

Conclusion

A lot of us grew up hating the word *discipline*. We equated browbeating, punishment, intentional embarrassment, shaming episodes, and put-downs with discipline. These harassments were actually delivered with the excuse that we were "being disciplined." We hope this chapter, which has discussed behavior critical to your success as both a clerk and a physician will help you and, if necessary, realign your own meanings for discipline. It is learning to use responsibility, delayed gratification, honesty, and balancing to further our lives, our work, and our relationships.

6 Getting Ready for Clerkships

Preparing for a clerkship has some parallels to getting ready for the "big" game or dance recital. Mental, physical, emotional, and spiritual preparations are all important. You'll need some knowledge, enough sleep, to be well fed, to be in good spirits, to be open to yourself and others, and to carry hopeful attitudes. You can't prepare for every circumstance, so work on the fundamentals: problem orientation, clear communication, how to connect with your patients, physical examination skills, and promptness.

Although you have already forgotten much of what you learned in Years 1 and 2, a lot of it stands by, waiting to be summoned. It will be easier to learn this time! But no matter how much you may recall from your basic science courses, *your evaluation will depend predominately on how you perform during the clerkship, not on the knowledge you bring with you.* **So affirm** (repeatedly, if necessary) "I'm here; I'll do my best. On clerkships I'll learn 90% of what I leave medical school with anyway."

A student, P.J., recalls anticipating his first major clerkship on pediatrics. He was fresh out of Year 2 plus a summer elective that provided opportunity to learn a number of skills:

> I was resolved to do well in the clerkships to improve my chances for a good internship. I was eager to prepare but not sure how to. Ten days before the clerkship began, I bought Nelson's text of pediatrics—the gold standard for peds. It weighed $10\frac{1}{2}$ pounds and had at least 2,000 pages. I had an intense summer and needed time off. How was I to use this book fruitfully in the short time I had to prepare? Answer—I wasn't. It was an impossible task. Graduates of the

peds clerkship had some good tips on learning to auscultate tiny hearts, restraining infants for ear exams, and urged memorizing infant nutrition and developmental "milestones" (favorite topics with the attendings). They neglected to tell me that peds is no friend to low back pain. No one suggested studying particular diseases ahead of time.

The following sections on knowledge, skills, and attitudes, discuss what you can do ahead of time to make your preparation fruitful.

Knowledge

Unless your medical school has a major commitment to problem-based learning, your courses in the first two years demanded robotlike memorization of massive volumes of material. However, this did teach you something: a vocabulary, a language, and how and where to look up material. Now you will need a more varied learning strategy. We recommend attention to the following points:

Be selective in the source of your learning materials. If issued a syllabus, read it. Otherwise, some students try to read the entire standard text. This is well nigh impossible and without a photographic memory is a waste of time. Some of P.J.'s colleagues on the pediatric clerkship read Nelson before the clerkship began. It was never apparent that they were better prepared.

It is instructive and fun to research a particular question in the journals, but most of your reading will be in one of the major texts and related to the problems of your patients. However, learning determined *exclusively* by your patients can lead to an inadequate knowledge base. You will be told (explicitly or implicitly), "Learn from your patients but also learn *all* of (medicine, surgery, etc.)." And indeed, you may be examined on "all," often through the use of NBME (National Board of Medical Examiners) shelf-copy exams (Chapter 12). Balance study based on patient contact with that based on the important clinical conditions addressed by the discipline. Table 6.1 lists high-priority, non-problem-oriented, knowledge and skills recommended for each particular specialty and three or more of the most common problems presenting to each major specialty clerkship. Review Table 6.1 with your clerkship director and faculty to identify changes or additional high-priority problems for your specific clerkship.

Table 6.1   Suggested Basic Study for Various Clerkships[a]

Specialty	Knowledge and Skills	Common Presenting Problems		
Pediatrics (outpatient)	Establishing rapport with kids	Diarrhea	Upper-respiratory infection	
Internal medicine	Interviewing patients EKG rhythms Physical & neurological exam AIDS precautions	Chest pain Abdominal mass Cerebrovascular accident	Chronic cough Diarrhea	Anemia Headache
Family practice (outpatient)	Interviewing Diagnosis & treatment of injuries & fractures; suturing	Low back pain Abnormal uterine bleeding	Cough and shortness of breath Upper-respiratory infection	Anxiety Alcohol abuse & dependence
Psychiatry	Interviewing Mental status exam	Hallucinations Suicidality	Depression	Aggressive behavior Anxiety
OB-GYN	Pelvic and breast exam Menstrual history	High-risk pregnancy Abnormal pap smear	Abnormal uterine bleeding	Menopausal symptoms
Critical care	EKG rhythms; CPR Critical neurological signs Diagnosis of internal bleeding	Chest pain Trauma with blood loss Shock	Head injury	Compound fractures Respiratory failure
Surgery	Postop fluid balance; suturing; dressing changes	Abdominal pain Traumatic injuries	Mass in breast	GI bleeding

a. Inpatient except where indicated.

45

Learn which problems, in your specialty, need to be on instant recall so that diagnosis and management can proceed promptly. This will happen as you accumulate experience. Be assured, in a critical situation, no one at your level can function with the precision and speed of the fictitious medical personnel portrayed on television. Only repetitive experience with a particular condition, followed by reflection will make you secure in the knowledge and skills required for emergencies. For nonemergency problems, you will have time to read, consult, or ask questions of the people who can help you. Seeing several examples of the same or similar clinical conditions will clarify abstract principles and add to your knowledge base.

Familiarize yourself with how the more common conditions in this specialty reveal themselves. Focus on the points that will differentiate one etiology from another in a particular patient. This will help you retain the knowledge and help the patient. For example, in internal medicine, myocardial infarction (MI) typically appears as "crushing" anterior chest pain. Infectious mono presents as sore throat, headache, and lymph node enlargement. Gall bladder disease most commonly gives right upper-abdominal pain or pain and fever.

Some major texts devote sections to problems in addition to those on each organ system. So in an internal medicine text, you can find discussions of abdominal pain, chest pain, diarrhea, cough, weight loss, and other problems. Skimming those will give you an idea of the range of possibilities that each represents.

For example, a 52-year-old hypertensive male presents with chest pain of unknown cause. To learn about chest pain, you could read about various *diseases* of the chest wall, *diseases* of the heart, and *diseases* of the respiratory system. You would discover that some of these diseases don't even cause chest pain. Alternatively, in the problem-oriented approach, you would key your reading to the problem of chest pain, quickly learning the various possibilities (such as MI [heart attack], pleurisy, and chest wall inflammation or injury) and how to tell them apart.

Read and study something related to each patient's main problem(s)—the principal reason(s) for seeking care. New patients don't show up with a disease (although they may have one); they show up with problems (a symptom, sign, or abnormal test result). The most frequent ones will vary, depending on patient mix and other factors.

Inpatient pediatrics (not shown in table) usually includes more rare diseases ("zebras"), and/or, in some hospitals, frequent cases of HIV-AIDS, oncology, and intensive care of premature infants. The inpatient family practice clerkship, where it exists, will be a mixture of problems seen in other inpatient clerkships.

The most frequent problems in outpatient clerkships can differ from those for inpatients in the same specialty. Thus, outpatient internal medicine has less critical care, more chronic long-term problems (diabetes, arthritis, overweight), and many periodic checkup and health maintenance visits. In outpatient surgery, postop care, outpatient (mostly minor) surgery, and evaluations for possible major surgery occupy the majority of the visits. Outpatient OB-GYN sees many periodic pelvic/Pap/breast exams, as well as cases of infertility, dysmenorrhea, and abnormal uterine bleeding. Outpatient psychiatry (depending on the venue) will be replete with anxiety, depression, adjustment disorders, anger management, and only a rare psychotic patient.

Hidden Problems

On all services be alert for the following "hidden" problems:

- Type II (adult onset) diabetes
- Early chronic obstructive pulmonary disease
- Anemia
- Depression
- Alcoholism or other drug abuse/dependence
- Physical and emotional abuse
- Unresolved grieving and loss: related to loved ones, jobs, places, capabilities, lifestyle
- Family tension, strife, and sick interpersonal dynamics

> **Cancer warnings:** abnormal bleeding, unexplained weight loss, unusual and continued pain, changing moles and other skin lesions, unexplained lumps and bumps, recent psychological changes, profound fatigue, low energy, unexplained anemia

Skills

Before your first clerkship, you acquired elemental skills in patient interviewing, physical examination, and organizing patient write-ups. Review these skills and look at habits you have acquired in relating to patients. Also, if the clerkship director does not assign you to write a learning plan for the clerkship, we suggest that you initiate one.

The most important skill to acquire, or sharpen, during any clerkship is the skill of self-education. It is a difficult process of monitoring yourself and honestly appraising your strengths and weaknesses (see Chapter 12, "Self-Examination"): For example, Do I really know how to listen reflectively? Am I present when I talk to patients? Unfortunately, self-evaluation is not explicitly emphasized in medical school.

Activity: List things that you are uncertain about. Write your responses to questions such as the following:

- How can I improve my approach to a patient from whom I must draw blood?
- What will I do if a patient gets angry?
- What scares me about the clerkship?
- What are some situations in which I might feel lost (e.g., your first code, a patient in shock, or one vomiting red blood).

The list will heighten self-awareness and help you learn by observing others in similar circumstances. You can ask about the frightening situations and learn how to prepare for them. *This activity increases the probability that you will observe and evaluate yourself—a skill that helps you improve all others.*

Do this self-diagnostic exercise in advance, because once you plunge into the frenzy of the clerkship, you may shut the questions off. The advance work can better equip you to handle the important issues.

Attitudes and
Personal Philosophy/Psychology

Your attitudes as you enter and participate in any clerkship are key determinants in the amount you learn and, quite probably, the grade you achieve.

Important attitudes include the following:

- I am the most important variable in determining what I learn in this clerkship.
- Whether or not this is a "good" clerkship, I can learn plenty.
- Clerkship education is much more than learning facts and concepts.
- Personality conflicts can diminish what I learn. I will avoid this possibility insofar as possible.
- This will be hard work, *and* I need to take good care of myself while the clerkship is in progress.

Several years ago we interviewed 56 second- and third-year medical students from seven different schools across the country. Those who manifested the first attitude listed above both had a better time and seemed to have learned more than the others. **So before clerkships begin, have an honest discussion with your best friend, partner, or therapist.** Look at how your attitudes, habitual reactions, stereotypes, and philosophical positions might affect what you want to achieve.

We do not advocate tailoring your political views or personal philosophy to be ingratiating, nor do we advocate avoiding conflict if it's a matter of important principle. We do urge being vigilant for attitudes that might unfavorably influence your experience.

Activity: Reflect on and write about each of the following:

- Think about how you deal with authority—in regard to parents, teachers, supervisors. Write about situations in which you experienced discomfort and/or conflict with an authority figure. Is there a pattern in your reactions (i.e., passive, passive-aggressive, confrontational)?
- What is your experience with sorrow and death?
- How do you react to strong and difficult feelings (anger, grief, frustration)?
- How do you think you will respond to stressful life-threatening emergencies?

Discussion of these and related questions with a "safe" person can reveal tripping stones to avoid.

Other Considerations

It will come as no surprise that good performance in the clinical setting is highly valued. Review "The Valued Clinical Clerk" (Box 5.1). Part II will advise you in detail how to perform well. Here are some "pregame" considerations that you will find helpful.

Competitiveness. Competitiveness is fostered by house staff, some faculty, and most grading systems. Be alert for it and don't collude with it. Some teachers will goad you by openly comparing student presentations: "Your colleague Jones made a superb presentation Tuesday. Hope you can do as well." Or they may "keep score" of answers to questions on rounds. Because performing well can influence your internship/residency placement, how will you deal with a fellow clerk who overtly undermines your work? Or with the one who is a slacker, thus making more work for you?

Dress and Paraphernalia. Plan to be neat and clean in grooming and dress. Neatness never offends. We like neckties on men. Scrub suits are fine, especially at night. But unless you're overwhelmed with work, change them when they are bloody or too rumpled. The white coat is required in many clerkships. We think they are a mistake on pediatrics and of minimal desirability elsewhere. They create distance more than they help rapport. The stethoscope is your most salient badge. *If you use it well as a diagnostic tool, its benefit as a status symbol is justified.*

On-Call Duty. Get a copy of the house staff call schedule so you know who is on-call. Also learn what conferences and rounds the house staff may attend off the unit.

Your Surroundings. Familiarize yourself with the layout of the unit and coordinate some of your daily routine to save unnecessary trips.

Find a quiet place. Some people can work anywhere. If you're lucky you'll find a peaceful nook on the unit or nearby. It might even be a place to nap when you are exhausted. In medical school, our friend Ben was a master at finding such spots. Many times, he spent the night in them—on-call or not!

Activity: Make sure both your resident and attending clarify the responsibilities they expect of you. It is better to do this with both of them at the same time. Questions might include the following:

- Do I attend all rounds; if not, which rounds?
- Is there a limit on the number of admissions I work up each week?
- What other duties do I have—such as drawing blood, transporting patients, checking on lab results?
- What irregular duties can I anticipate?
- Where can I keep a few belongings?

Part II

The Work and Challenges of Clerkship: The Journey Itself

7 Honoring the Patient

The relationship between physician and patient is a phenomenon as much a part of sickness and medicine as the diseases that make people sick. It makes a sick person into a patient and it makes a medical person into a doctor and a clinician. The most skillful practitioner raises the relationship to an art . . . negotiating between intimacy and separateness, between empathy and objectivity.

—Eric Cassell (1991, p. 79)

The patient is the expert on their own personal being and the physician must not forget that.

—Third-year medical student

Most students come to medical school because they "want to help people." By the time you get to clerkships—real medicine at last—the rigors of your studies and your impersonal treatment as a first- and second-year student may have dimmed your altruism. We join our colleague, Dr. Joseph Zarconi, in urging you to remember, "The patient is why I am here."

"To honor the patient" must be the overriding value of medical education and practice. On some clerkships, led by enlightened attendings, honoring is indeed a major consideration—although seldom explicit. Rarely does a teacher say both verbally and through modeling, "It is essential to honor your patients."

A prime goal of this chapter and book is to help you graduate from medical school habituated to honoring your patients. Our two subsequent chapters are devoted to communication (8) and the patient appraisal (9). Together, Chapters 7 through 9 will help you interact and communicate effectively and sensitively with your patients, teachers, and health care colleagues and to conduct comprehensive and effective data collection and management. *These skills/attributes are vital to the consummate practice of medicine.*

Honoring Your Patients:
Nine Principles

Have no illusions, honoring your patients is a big order, and often in busy, stressful situations, it's very difficult. As time passes, it will become more natural, but even with experience, it requires energy and time. Begin by learning to identify, avoid, and erase, *dishonoring behaviors,* such as breaking confidentiality, violating modesty, not answering questions, and several more that are inherent in the principles that follow. Many of the obstacles to communication discussed in Chapter 8 are also dishonoring behaviors.

Activity: Write down some of the ways that you honor your friends and family. Also, note some of the ways that you are neutral toward them or dishonor them.

Principle 1: The patient has primacy (not his or her doctor, not his or her disease) in the care process. A rational, uninformed person observing a busy practice might see the physician as the most important person involved, with nurses and others in the supporting cast. The observer would also identify disease (or injury) as the main focus of everyone's attention. The patient may be treated more like goods in transfer than a person who is ill, fearful, in pain, or suffering in other ways. You ask, "How does this become a problem since people become doctors to help others?" That's the paradox. Most students do learn to help people through the use of medications, surgery, diagnostic tests, and a variety of other treatments. But too often, *the dominant focus of medical education and training becomes diagnosis and treatment of disease rather than care of the patient.* Unfortunately, patients themselves often cooperate in this dynamic.

Patients should have top billing. With nurses and other caregivers, doctors need to hold the patient as the main focus of their attention.

Principle 2: Don't objectify the patient. When the disease has primacy, the patient is more readily objectified, ignored, or minimized. The *person* involved is neglected. "The doctors I trust most are those that either look up or remember some details, some little thing I have told them that is distinctive to me" (a patient).

Because people are different, the same *disease* (see glossary) in different persons results in very different *illnesses* (see glossary and Chapter 9). Illness acknowledges the person harboring the disease or injury, the effects of the disease on patient, family, job, and other aspects of life, and also recognizes aspects of the patient's lifestyle, social patterns, and family dynamics that contribute to his sickness. Thus, focusing on disease and not on illness contributes, sometimes in major ways, to objectification.

> A man in his 40s was hospitalized in shock due to extensive gastrointestinal bleeding. After he was stabilized, studies identified an active duodenal ulcer. Medical treatment was begun; he was named "the bleeder in 521." He fretted considerably about missing work and his wife's "greasy cooking." Despite this, team members focused solely on the pharmacology of H2 blockers. The impact of his condition on work, finances, and family was not their concern.

This man was treated like an *embodied disease*, not a person. In contrast—

> A 40-year-old woman had an acute, severe flare-up of previously mild rheumatoid arthritis. With her input, doctors considered how this flare-up and its sequelae might effect her job, spousal and parent-child relationships, ability to exercise, feelings of self-esteem, and her bank account. Her sense of value and worth was honored; the team attended to her *illness*.

Labeling also objectifies (see also Chapter 8). The following statements from a third-year student is illustrative:

> A student says to his colleague: "My new patient is just another history and physical—angina, just plain old angina, you know how boring that is. It's a great case for a P-Dog (second-year student learning physical diagnosis). This is an easy hit for me. . . . She'll be gone Thursday unless something happens . . . but this'll be a good EKG."

Implicit here is the attitude, that since this new patient has the same disease as others, the work will be the same.

Principle 3: Integrate the patient's emotional and spiritual concerns into the diagnosis and management plan. To do this, you must tune into such concerns, truly hear what is said, and then integrate them into your communication with the patient. The patient's story is usually a cognitive declaration nuanced to varying degrees with emotion. The exam seeks physical findings. The physician's manner of discussing these findings and reporting the lab data and treatment plan is habitually cognitive and often neglects the emotional and spiritual domains entirely. If, in neuroanatomy, you were told, "Forget about the white matter; learn only the gray structures," you would not fully appreciate the complexity and sophistication of the brain.

The bottom line is this: *We can cure or ameliorate disease and injury, sometimes dramatically, but if, at the same time, the minds, emotions, and spirits of patients are not greeted and nurtured they will not be honored or feel satisfied.*

Principle 4: Show respect. *Observe confidentiality,* a key facilitator in the patient-physician relationship. Doctors and nurses threaten confidentiality by discussing patients in a hallway or elevator. This is bad practice even if the patient's name is not mentioned.

> While attending a social gathering, a physician colleague overheard an internist telling another guest about a patient our colleague had seen in consultation. The internist used the patient's name—a gross violation of confidentiality.

Break confidentiality and you promptly dishonor the patient.

Respect the patient's modesty and privacy. The patient deserves physical privacy: During your exam and during rounds, pull the curtains around the bed if he or she is not in a private room. Unless assisting the patient, don't approach the bedside if he or she is on the bedpan or using the urinal. Before removing blankets and sheets covering the patient, explain the need.

Honoring the patient may include touching appropriately. There are many times when it is appropriate and helpful to hold a patient's hand, place your hand on an arm or shoulder, or put your arm around him or her. There are times when a hug is appropriate—*but always ask first.*

Explain what you're doing. This is particularly important when you are embarking on a procedure unfamiliar to the patient.

Data are patient's property. This includes the patient narrative and history, the physical examination, and lab tests. He or she has a right to know what is found, what we deem important, and how we interpret it. The patient has a right to a copy of his or her medical record.

Don't rush. Although your time is limited, rushing devalues the patient. It is critical to be unhurried and considerate during the interview—wherein you glean intimate knowledge—and the physical exam, as you touch and move the patient who is partially or completely unclothed. Physicians adept at gaining rapport seem unhurried even when they spend only a few minutes in the room.

Elsewhere, we outline the collaborative partnership. The patient and the caregiver work as a team (Ways, 1985, pp. 161-162). This is the ultimate in respecting the patient as an adult person, not treating him or her as a child or an object. Not all patients or physicians will undertake this kind of partnership, but the rewards are significant for those who do.

Principle 5: Strive for clear communication (also see Chapters 8 and 9). *Listen attentively* to hear patients' needs, values, fears, desires, and especially to encourage their stories to unfold. Investigate patients' attitudes about illness (why they are ill, is there meaning to their illness), their capacity for self-care, and what and how much they want done.

A physician found a rectal mass, almost certainly cancer, in a 58-year-old man. The surgeons advised removal; this was refused despite a clear explanation on the consequences of delay. Two years later, the tumor had not enlarged or otherwise changed. Lab tests and X-rays showed no evidence of metastasis.

Be receptive and open to the individual's fears, anger, and other concerns. We pay more attention to this with new patients; we need their history to proceed effectively. Later in the relationship, we may not be as attentive to this.

Always keep the patient informed, and when a severely ill patient is referred to a specialist, stay in contact.

One 76-year-old woman with long-standing rheumatoid arthritis was referred to a GI specialist by her primary care physician and her rheumatologist, who suspected a "stomach problem." A malignancy of the stomach was diagnosed, and total gastrectomy was performed. Three weeks later, she saw an oncologist and began chemotherapy. Eight more weeks had passed when the patient stated, perplexed, that neither her primary care physician nor her rheumatologist had called.

This patient's technical care could not be faulted, but she felt abandoned by the physicians she had seen regularly over the prior decade.

Use language the patient can understand. It is rude to use abbreviations with the patient. They are a foreign language and make the patient feel more isolated. If abbreviations are used by others on rounds, translate for the patient before leaving his or her bedside.

Answer the patient's questions. If you can't or don't have time to answer, it's OK to say, "That's an important question, but now is not a good time for me." Or, "There are a couple of things I need to get done before talking to you. I'll come back around seven and we'll discuss your question." The patient feels acknowledged and attended to.

Principle 6: Be genuine and honest in manner, speech, and spirit. *"Doctor and patient are bound in a reciprocal relationship* [italics added]—failure to understand that is failure to comprehend clinical medicine" (Cassell, 1991, p. 76). Sincerity and honesty are essential to achieving a "bound" relationship. They are pillars of genuineness—fertilizing trust and helping to ensure a meaningful connection. Say you don't know when you don't, and get help if and when you need it. Be honest about the facts of the case, and when you're not sure how to do that, ask for help from someone more experienced. Don't pretend to be something you aren't. While still a student, designating yourself as doctor is an unhelpful subterfuge. It may comfort you, but it is unnecessary and may backfire. Introduce yourself as a student doctor or a medical student.

Being genuine also requires honesty about your own emotions. It is useful to reveal something about yourself, but such openness must be responsible. Answer the question, "How are you?" with reality, not just the shopworn "Fine." If you're discouraged, it's OK to say that. If can be OK to say you've been irritated or angry without mentioning specific names or circumstances. Some of your pleasures can be revealed. To talk extensively about your own problems is inappropriate and can give an excuse for the patient to deflect or control the interview, but some personal vulnerability demonstrates that you are a person too, not only a student or caregiver, and this will strengthen rapport: "I'm pretty tired." "I am feeling rushed today." "You remind me of my grandfather."

It is not OK to complain to the patient that you are overworked or that you're very annoyed with the surgical consult or to discuss your finances or sex life.

We are not in the doctor-patient relationship to have our own emotional needs met.

Insincere reassurance is a barrier to effective communication. Compliments and positive remarks are helpful if they are sincere, not spoken to cheer a patient on false or tenuous grounds. Remember that sick people are more vulnerable in general. Often, even the ballyhooed "bedside manner" is counterfeit, a facade. Indeed, Bolton (1979, p. 260) points out that the word *personality* is derived from the Latin *persona,* an actor's mask!

Principle 7: Be empathetic. Empathy is experiencing another's feelings while preserving your own identity—an "accurate response to another's needs without being infected by them" (Bolton, 1979, p. 271).

Empathy involves three processes: understanding the other's feelings, comprehension of what precipitated those feelings, and communication that helps the other person feel accepted and understood. Ask yourself, "How does he or she feel while saying/doing this?" *Empathy is critical to a maturing patient-doctor relationship.*

Antipathy—apathy—sympathy—empathy are on a continuum. Antipathy is aversion. Antipathy toward a patient, as opposed to something he or she may have done, is serious. If it cannot be reversed or mitigated, transfer responsibility to another caregiver. This honors both your feelings and the patient's welfare.

Apathy is the absence of feeling. "Apathy, when it is prevalent in significant relationships, can be very destructive" (Bolton, 1979, p. 271). It is sometimes confused with sympathy. Sympathy is a feeling *for* rather than *with* (empathy) someone. Depending on how it is delivered, it can be condescending with connotations of "poor thing." We need more empathy cards, fewer sympathy cards! "Consistent undiluted sympathy, I believe, is even more harmful than apathy" (Bolton, 1979, p. 271).

The tendency in medicine has been for providers to move toward apathy with an attitude of "detached concern" (Lief & Fox, 1963) and/or to the side of sympathy with a facile or jaded bedside manner. Neither serves to foster a healthy and useful relationship between doctor and patient.

Activity: Imagine yourself as one of your own patients. How do you feel? How would you cope with his or her situation? Does this differ from what the actual patient feels or will do?

Empathy helps us to be aware of and acknowledge a patient's suffering. It is difficult to overlook a patient's physical pain, but frequently, we overlook the many other ways that patients suffer—often more deeply than with physical pain. The threat of death or disability, loss of identity, forced idleness, and loss of control over life are among the common causes of suffering (see Chapter 19).

Finally, we acknowledge that empathy is difficult—particularly with people you don't know well or those from backgrounds different from your own. True empathy may not always be possible, particularly on brief exposure to the patient. However, avoiding antipathy, apathy, and sympathy is not so hard.

Principle 8: Be willing to extend yourself for the patient's betterment. "Be willing" conveys both intention and action. It is "not an emotional sentiment of liking, nor romantic attraction, . . . nor yet an intellectual attitude," but "the will of the self in devotion to the neighbor." (Beach & Niebuhr, 1955, quoted in Bolton, 1979, p. 263). It is also akin to Buber's (1958) "the responsibility of an *I* for a *Thou.*" (p. 14). In the following story, the student knew her help was needed even though a powerful consultant had predicted the patient's imminent demise.

> Sally Ryan, a fourth-year student, admitted a 42-year-old man with acute pancreatitis at midday. The patient suffered severe pain and persistent vomiting, and his blood pressure and serum calcium were dangerously low. The head of the GI service, a brilliant and feared attending made an extra trip across town to see the man that same day. After examining the patient and checking the vital signs and lab results, he predicted, without hesitation, a fatal outcome before morning. That night, the ward nurses were short-staffed, and the intern had several new patients. The man with pancreatitis needed constant regulation of intravenous medication to sustain his blood pressure. Ryan spent her night off at the patient's bedside monitoring blood pressure and other signs and regulating the flow of IV meds. At daylight, the patient sat up in bed, shook the student's hand and said, "Thank you. I'm going to make it." He went on to complete recovery. The GI attending graciously disclosed both his amazement and appreciation.

Willingness to extend oneself for the betterment of the patient makes medicine tricky. How far and how often can you extend yourself without damaging yourself and your relationships? It is an issue of balance (see Chapter 5).

This is discussed further in the chapters on exhaustion (13) and self-care (17 and 18).

Principle 9: Be accepting and nonjudgmental. Finally, honoring the patient must involve the ability to *accept people as they are, no matter what you think of their behavior, their likes and dislikes, or their beliefs.* A patient's actions may be unhelpful or unhealthy, but this does not make him or her or a bad person.

Do your best to not judge a person as right or wrong.

Over years, a specialist in chemical dependency interviewed and examined several individuals who classified themselves as "bums" at one time in their lives. Severely addicted to alcohol and or other drugs, each one had been, by their own admission, one or more of the following: a derelict, dishonest, criminal, abusive, manipulative, abjectly dependent. They are now healthy and productive for many years since becoming clean and sober.

Don't make snap judgments. This is difficult with some patients—homeless people, addicts, the angry person, the overtly dependent and frightened, and the powerful personality that manifests impatience, aggressiveness, or both. One of us watched the following scenario.

A man was admitted with a new myocardial infarction (MI). The resident arrived at the bedside to insert a central venous pressure line. Still in some pain, the patient was restless and moved his arm as the procedure was beginning. "Hold still, you ___hole," said the resident. The patient had a cardiac arrest. Cardiopulmonary resuscitation was unsuccessful. He died!

A harsh judgment was made and felt. In all likelihood it triggered the patient's sudden demise.

Do not contaminate the interpersonal environment with evaluations/judgments of the patients' feelings, thoughts, and behaviors. Even if you do not like certain aspects of the way your patient lives his or her life, you can still treat and honor him or her as a person. A social outcast or a participant in shady business dealings is still a person. A patient may talk too much; he or she is still a person. He or she may be abusive and manipulative—two characteristics that are the stepchildren of insecurity and low self-esteem; the patient is still a person. *Keep looking and listening for the genuine core qualities of your patient.*

Activity: Make up a brief four- to five-item rating scale for honoring the patient using this chapter as a guide. Rate yourself on five consecutive patients to whom you are assigned for a minimum of three days.

A Paradox

Although we urge you to honor the patient, you may not be truly honored in your role as student. Prior to clerkships, you have been more like one of a herd than an individual. Your emotional sensitivities have been largely ignored (see Chapter 16), your intellect eroded (see Chapter 15), and your valuable relationships strained and perhaps broken. So now we tell you to honor the patient! Treat the patient in the ways you would like to be treated as a student. What irony!

Resolution of this paradox lies partly in the fact that, in contrast to the first two years, *your experience of a clerkship can be different from many learning experiences that preceded it in medical school.* Although many of the herd perspectives seen in science faculty also operate among your clinical teachers, they are less prominent and in some teachers, even absent. You will have some recognition as an individual. With initiative, you will have the opportunity to use your mind in critical and creative ways, and with work, you can come to some state of familiarity and peace with the feelings stimulated by the stark human dramas that unfold before you.

8 Communication

[The] Hippocratic school based its diagnosis and treatment on objective measurement. . . . it decidedly did not include much of what the patient said, since that was merely opinion. Thus, Virgil called medicine "the silent art."

—*Eric Cassell (1976, p. 56)*

The language and technology of medical communication have changed considerably in the last 30 to 40 years. Charts and medical talk are replete with a "shorthand alphabet soup of letters and numbers." Sophisticated and valuable diagnostic tests combined with increasing use of computers have significantly eroded use of the patient narrative and atrophied our skills in physical examination. Lowenstein (1997) ventures that "the transformation of language cuts off all but the most pragmatic and immediate communication between students of medicine and their teachers or mentors . . . and affects the process of role modeling, which is a critical part of the physician's development." The indictment deepens as he states that the "increasingly apparent gap" between patients and their doctors also derives in part from the same changes in language and paradigms. Our cry for the doctors of our childhood is "but a yearning for communication in a common language . . . [including] a great number of terms for hope, reassurance, strength, and courage" (p. 22)

Quality patient care and management depend on good communication and teamwork. Communication also lies at the core of accomplished learning, powerfully influences patient satisfaction, and is the life blood of healthy relationships. This chapter outlines a basic model of communication for your work with patients, teachers, and other caregivers. It defines common barriers to good communication with patients, colleagues, and people in our personal lives.

Activity: For a day, watch the interactions between residents, nurses, students, and attendings.

- What barriers do you observe between people or categories?
- What suggestions might you make to two or more of the people involved?
- Talk with a friend about any prior experiences that remind you of being in this clerkship. (A previous clerkship does not qualify.)
- What changes in your own communication style might make you more effective?

Overview of Health Care Communication

Figure 8.1 illustrates the complexities of hospital/clinic communication. It is a difficult diagram to look at and comprehend—which is exactly the point. Any clerkship involves you, the patients, your residents and attending, the nursing staff, and other health professionals in an amalgam of relationships. The caregiver-patient relationship is central to the patient care process, and in the hospital, 20 to 30 roles involving two or more hospital departments support any given patient. His transfer to another service can double these figures. The pathways by which orders, diagnostic requests (lab, X-ray, etc.), referrals, and consultations move are complex (Figure 8.2). Outpatient settings can also be complicated; teamwork and good communication are no less essential.

A Model for Communication

The Basic Model

Sending. In addition to being *clear,* quality messages must be *concise* and *clean* (honest)—the *three Cs. A sender is clear when he or she knows what he or she wants to convey and says or writes that in understandable language.* To attain

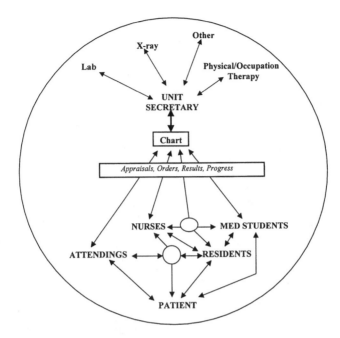

Figure 8.1. Communication Pathways in Patient Care

clarity, try again if it feels like you're not getting through. Don't assume you are always clear. Monitor this intermittently: "What did you hear me say?" The glossary of terms at the end of the book helps you to understand certain words in the way we want them understood.

Be as concise as you can. Stick to your goal and the subject. Don't sidetrack.

Communication is clean when both the sender and the receiver exclude emotional or political baggage; defensiveness or competitiveness is an example. This is often difficult. Your tone of voice, the words you choose, and your body language can all project judgments, blame, and opinions that may put off the listener.

Receiving/Listening. Listening is at the heart of quality relationships. It is difficult to listen well. One can easily misinterpret a message. Here's an example:

After one student had been on the clerkship a week, his resident said in a stern tone, "You need to be here on time for rounds every day." Another resident nearby interpreted this as, "We're not sure you are

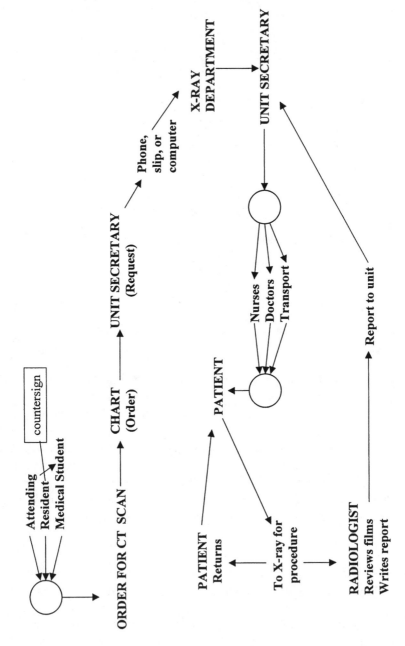

Figure 8.2. The Pathway of an Order for a CT Scan

as motivated as we would like." The student however, told his adviser, "They really think I'm doing badly—I might flunk."

As a receiver, pay attention and listen reflectively. Don't think about how you will respond or interrupt prematurely ("walk on the others words"). Reflective listening does not approve/disapprove, advise, criticize, interpret, or remain completely silent. A reflective listener makes a good guess about the speaker's meaning and then checks it out. "Are you worried about child care for your grandchild while you're in the hospital?" Asking the right questions is a very important function of the good receiver.

The Channel. The channel is the space through which the message must travel—across the room, through the telephone wire, via an Internet server or a relay station. *When relaying a message from one person to another, you are the channel.* During conversation, noise, interruptions, or other distractions (static!) clog the channel. You clear the channel by lessening extraneous noise and distractions. Pulling curtains around the bed or closing the door of a patient's room can greatly improve communication.

Emphasis on Honesty

Honesty is important in both sending and receiving—including honesty about emotions. Contrast the following situations. In both, an important lab test wasn't done. The first attending said, caustically, "It's pretty sad this wasn't done. When my mother was in the hospital recently, somebody forgot to check her prothrombin time. As a result, she had GI bleeding that required transfusion." An emotionally charged event from the attending's past distorted his response to the situation. The other attending said, "It is important that we have that lab test done. Please order it STAT and I'll sign the slip." Later, he offered suggestions to the student about keeping track of important details.

We won't be effective and clear with others if we are dishonest with ourselves. *Without intellectual and emotional honesty, quality communication cannot occur.* If you want to leave work early because your Dad's visiting town but harbor irritation or anger over scut work, it will be difficult to ask for time off until you clear the air. You may need to talk with yourself in the mirror, walk with a friend, or ventilate to a confidant over the phone. If you feel safe doing so, it is best to calmly acknowledge your feelings to the resident.

Although not easy, such directness is usually possible. Many students fear that candor about feelings will jeopardize their evaluations. In a particular situation, if your gut tells you it might be a mistake, then don't do it. But calm and honest confession of feelings often leads to a fruitful discussion of what went on, heightened cooperation, and sometimes increased camaraderie. If communication is mutually respectful, the outcome can be positive for both parties.

> Sophia was on a clerkship in internal medicine. Her morning commute took one hour, and the clerkship director had emphasized punctuality for 7:30 a.m. work rounds. During her first week, one resident was consistently 15 to 25 minutes late. Sophia, sleep deprived in any case, seethed. Her presentations suffered. She delayed responding to requests made by the offending resident. He, in turn, became angry at her. Two weeks went by before Sophia stated her anger to the attending and the resident.

Some Refinements Through Transactional Analysis

Transactional analysis (TA) adds another dimension to the basic model. TA stipulates that any adult may communicate from the stance of a child, a parent, or an adult. The *child* wants to please and can't act independently or make mature decisions. The *parent* is authoritarian, opinionated, protective, and needs to be in control. A person may not modify or abandon the parental stance in favor of the adult one even when it would be clearly beneficial. Mature in actions and words, the *adult* expresses his or her own values and convictions but willingly listens to what others advocate, need, and want. The adult can alter his or her approach for a better alternative without loss of self-esteem.

In the workplace, mature people work to communicate in the *adult-adult* mode, using appropriate language and vocabulary and listening carefully and respectfully to one another. They will check out potential misunderstandings and repeat statements if they are not understood.

On a busy service, however, the faculty-staff hierarchy, and parental posturing in many teaching-patient care situations, makes adult-adult interaction inconstant. There is a lot going on—emergencies and other intense activities. When people are strained, they can react in a parental or childish mode rather than an adult one. So on clerkships, attending staff-resident-student dynamics may mirror family-of-origin issues (which stick to us like glue) for one or more of the players. Students may be treated like children. They may adopt the hero role and continually work to please. In an emergency, a faculty member or a fearful student may alter an established adult-adult relationship to a parent-child situation that is not as effective.

Residents and attendings often relate to students the way they do with patients. When the doctor-patient pattern is parent-child, the physician may also treat students as children. If their attending is bored with patients, students will read that into the attending's attitudes toward them. The "proportionality" shown in the box illustrates this:

Doctor : Teacher   Consciously or unconsciously,
Patient : Student   students may perceive a parallel between the caregiver-patient dynamic and what they experience between themselves and the teacher.

A student may then adopt behavior that reinforces the parent-child pattern by either trying to please or by acting out—perhaps by doing the scut work slowly.

The ideal, of course, is consistent adult-adult behavior in both the physician-patient and teacher-student relationships.

Obstacles to Communication

Five major obstacles to high-quality communication are judging, sending solutions ("fixing"), avoiding the other's concerns, talking another language, and playing games.

Judging

Differentiate how you feel about a behavior from how you feel about the person. An overweight cardiac patient describes three months of florid dietary indiscretion. He is not "bad"; this is unhealthy behavior on the part of a good person. If you can make this distinction clear, he need not feel rejection. Your "emotional bank account" (see Covey, 1989, pp. 188-202) will be intact. It is unquestionably difficult to maintain an attitude of acceptance in the face of a life-endangering addiction or child abuse, but **your task is to stay in relationship with a patient even when you deplore his or her behavior.**

Criticizing is a common way of judging. Physicians commonly criticize addicts, overweight people, and smokers. "Mr. Stewart, this is ridiculous; it's bad for you to smoke, you should have stopped long ago." It is more effective to just give the evidence ("smokers are at far greater risk for lung cancer, emphysema, and heart disease . . ."). If patients ask for your opinion, give it, but don't alienate your patient with personal criticism.

Labeling is troublesome. We all use labels as shorthand in perfectly acceptable ways("she's a go-getter"), but their use in health care is problematic. Residents say, "The 'cardiac' in 121 needs water," or "Let's see the 'wheezer' next and then the 'whiner.' " This depersonalizes and objectifies patients (Chapter 7). Labeling or speaking of someone as "a victim" may influence their reaction to illness or lead to serious self-devaluation.

Some professionals use an otherwise legitimate diagnostic label too early or too often. They listen to part of someone's story, hear a salient cue, then immediately voice a diagnosis or label. This happens often with psychological-behavioral disorders such as depression, perpetual victim, substance abuse, and borderline personality. The label then becomes the frame of reference.

Cueing into the diagnosis or label is important in the diagnostic process. Premature use of it before adequate supporting data has been obtained or inappropriate expression of it in front of the patient can be harmful. Labeling in these ways is disrespectful and can become a pernicious and damaging habit.

Before bringing her into the room, the student presented a new outpatient. The woman, 34, had chronic neck pain attributed to an auto accident one year earlier. She had sought care in three other clinics but complained that "they didn't listen to me," "wouldn't give me enough time," and, "I disagreed with the nurse practitioner about ibuprofen." At this point, the attending, an internist competent in psychosocial disorders, said confidently, "Sounds borderline." When the patient came in, the attending examined her, assuming that the neck pain was secondary to an injury and her troubles with caregivers due to a "borderline personality." The team referred her to PT. A week later, she had a seizure and exhibited neurological signs that the physicians had not attempted to elicit during her first visit. Further tests identified a nonmalignant brain tumor. Surgery was successful, and she recovered uneventfully. In retrospect, the personality "aberrations" had actually been observed by family before the auto accident.

This is a dramatic example of how labeling—even using medical terminology—can be a disservice to the patient.

You ask, "Is labeling OK if you don't do it in front of the patient?" Labeling often has its roots in expediency and/or disrespect. **Regard labeling as a warning to yourself. It is time to look at your feelings about the patient(s) and your work.**

"Fixing" or Sending Solutions

Liberal use of antibiotics for upper-respiratory infection (URI) is a classic example of fixing. Most URIs are viral. Few viruses respond to antibiotics. Often, the patient provokes such a solution, and the physician is an informed accomplice. The physician can also initiate fixing—"I advise you to try this medication"—without explanations or alternatives. The patient is not involved in the decision. *The goal is to involve the patient so that orders and prescriptions are the logical outcome of considered dialogue.* For example, "We might consider felodipine for your fingers. Have you heard of it? Do you know what it does? Here's how it works. . . ."

Avoiding Patient's Concerns

Excessive or inappropriate reassurance avoids or minimizes patients' concerns. It can be a form of emotional withdrawal or a put-down. "Reassurance is often used by people who like the idea of being helpful but who do not want to experience the emotional demand that goes with it" (Bolton, 1979, p. 25).

Using excessive logic or explanation is not helpful. Most sick people can't process a lot of facts. Also, logic can avoid feelings that, in turn, reflect concerns.

Diverting or discounting devalues patients and their concerns. If you say, "Well I hear your concern, Mrs. Zalinsky, but let's talk about your smoking," she feels devalued or stupid. What matters to the patient doesn't matter to you.

Humor delivered from a loving stance (which is often hard to do) can strengthen rapport. Light humor that is kind and harmless can aid communication, help release tension, and cheer the patient. Humor directed at the patient's infirmity or shortcomings, even if the patient shrugs it off, will lessen trust. Harsh, vindictive humor is damaging under any circumstances. Frequently, too, a humorous remark can hide fear or repulsion. **Be aware of using humor as a shield.**

Talking (and Writing) Another Language

Abbreviations (including diagnostic ones such as COPD for chronic obstructive pulmonary disease) and jargon are two-edged swords. They can streamline communication, but they may bewilder or offend the patient. We favor sparse use of verbal abbreviations. Written abbreviations should be drawn from a clearly posted lexicon or glossary (the glossary at the end of this book is an example).

Frequent, unfamiliar, or ambiguous abbreviations may lead to errors. A social worker told us, "I hate to read charts. I feel stupid—out of the loop. Sometimes even the nursing staff can't translate for me."

Equally serious, during bedside or office discussions, patients in unfamiliar surroundings may feel like they are in a foreign country. Box 8.1 gives excerpts from an overabbreviated presentation. The problem list is all shorthand for diagnostic labels. Before they are used in front of the patient, he should be told in unabbreviated language what his problems are.

As well as its effects on the patient, *use of abbreviations also draws the house staff, students, and attendings further into their own world where they insulate more easily from the emotional and social concerns of the patient, other staff, and from their own feelings.* Even if abbreviations have not been used directly in front of them, a patient may intuit the distancing and expediency that underlies their use.

Activity: For one day don't use verbal or written abbreviations.

Responding to
Specific Situations for Your Patient(s)

Early in any clerkship, you may be assigned a few patients that "belonged" to students who have left the service. These people may be discharged, transferred, or enter a crisis before you come to know them. Listed below are two or three possible comments for each of several common situations. One or more of them may be appropriate.

Impending discharge:

• How do you feel about the possibility of going home?

BOX 8.1

Excerpts From a Presentation of Mr. Bryant

From Physical Exam
Heart: LBCD 14CM L MSL, 6th ICS, PMI 12 cm L MSL 5th ICS, S3 G,
no *m*

Neuro: DTR's symet., FNF, HTS, RAM all WNL
Problem List:

1. CHF 2° ASCVD
2. COPD
3. AODM
4. UTI

- You've improved a lot in the last few days (or your lab tests and clinical condition have stabilized); we feel you are ready to go home.

Transfer (or possible transfer) to another service:

- Well, Mr. Tracy, your pneumonia has cleared, and all your tests and vital signs are stable. So we've asked the eye doctors to consider taking care of your cataract before sending you home.
- Well, Sir, your diabetes has stabilized, and the surgeons are ready to operate on your colon, so you'll be moving up to surgery today.

Apprehension about a family visit:

- What feelings are you having about your family meeting (. . . Dad's visit, . . . seeing your son again) today?
- When your wife and kids come today, we'll explore their feelings about your drinking. It won't be easy for you, but it could be very important for your sobriety.

Bad news about diagnosis, tests, progress:

- Your test results are back, and the news is not what we would have liked to hear; here's the story: . . .
- The medicine (or procedure) is not working as well as we'd hoped. Let's talk about what that may mean and what other options we have.

Hopelessness or depression:

- You seem pretty sad. Can you talk with me about it?
- Depression can be powerful and clever. It often denies itself and makes us stubborn about seeking help. Counseling might benefit you, and for some depressions good medication is available. We will discuss your situation on rounds, and Dr. Smith or I will tell you our recommendations.

The patient knows he or she is dying and the end is near:

Statements here vary greatly depending on how long the outcome has been clear and what the patient has done to prepare for death.

- Is there anyone in particular that you want to talk with (. . . have visit) or that might help you at this time in any way?
- How can I be of help or comfort to you at this point?

The patient has metastatic cancer and is in severe, unremitting pain:

- We will keep you as comfortable as possible. There are ways to do that in which you control your own pain medication.
- I know you are feeling severe pain. I do not have the experience to recommend a particular course of treatment. I will ask my resident and attending to see you as soon as possible.

Activity: Memorize one response from three or more of the above categories. Role-play some of the situations with a colleague or friend. Switch roles. These activities will help you get a feel for the actual circumstances.

Students' Responsibility for Good Communication

You must assume significant responsibility for achieving good communication with patients and team members. If you want your job relationships to work (rather than blaming others when they don't work), you must do your part in enhancing communication. This is usually well received by faculty members even when they are very busy. Follow the suggestions given in this chapter and avoid the "obstacles to communication." Keep your communication intellectually and emotionally honest.

9 The Patient Appraisal

Each person carries his own doctor inside him. They come to us not knowing the truth. We are at our best when we give the doctor who resides within each patient a chance to go to work.

—Attributed to Albert Schweitzer

Despite our generally discouraging opinions of the educational process in medicine, we regard the clerkship experience and particularly the patient appraisal as a unique, exciting, and gratifying educational phenomenon. It has parallels to apprenticeship in the trades but is more physically and emotionally demanding and generally more rigorous.

In carrying out a patient appraisal, you have the experience of interviewing and examining a patient, adding other data if available, then formulating your own ideas of what is happening with the patient and what should be done. Shortly thereafter (sometimes almost simultaneously), *more experienced people are engaged in making a patient appraisal. You can compare your work and thinking with theirs almost immediately.* Then others, with even more experience, make comments and guide the team in the formulation of plans for further diagnosis and treatment (including, sometimes, the choice of doing nothing). An armamentarium of diagnostic procedures and interventions is on hand. Experts on special facets of the patient's problem complex are available for consultation. It is hard to fault this process as an exemplary learning strategy.

Importance of the Patient Appraisal

The patient appraisal is the heart and soul of the patient care process. Without it, nothing proceeds. The quality patient appraisal requires certain attitudes, discipline, and high-fidelity communication. Thus, this chapter follows logically from those preceding it: Chapter 5, "The Discipline of Patient Care"; Chapter 7, "Honoring the Patient" (the cardinal discipline of patient care); and Chapter 8, "Communication." Here, we lay out the guidelines and skills of the appraisal.

The following diagram depicts the essential elements of the medical/patient care process.

Patient Appraisal → Intervention(s) → Progress/Outcomes

The main steps of the patient appraisal are these:

1. **Data collection,** which gives rise to the *database* (see Box 9.1)
2. **Problem formulation,** giving rise to the *problem list*
3. **Assessment** (your thinking), recorded as *assessment(s)*
4. **Plan(s)** (for diagnostic and therapeutic interventions), recorded as *plan(s)*

The assessment(s) and plan(s) are recorded for each major active problem separately or in various combinations).[1] Progress and outcomes keyed to one or more problems are recorded in the *progress notes.*

Sources of Data and Their Organization in the Chart

Table 9.1 illustrates how the various sources contribute to the database as conventionally organized in the chart. The database of the patient appraisal is organized as shown in the left-hand column. The most common sources of data (interviews, preexisting data, exams, diagnostic tests) are across the top and their relative contribution to each section is indicated in the cells. The patient interview, physical exam (PE), old records, and basic lab data usually provide the most crucial information. They reveal most of what the patient and his or her previous caregivers know about the present illness (major active problem[s]).

BOX 9.1

Organization of Database

The *chief complaint or presenting circumstances* is the leading entry in the recorded patient appraisal and needs no explanation.

Patient profile is a sketch of the patient's personality; it characterizes his or her relationships to immediate family and close friends. It describes the patient's relationship to work, hobbies, amusements, spiritual/religious beliefs and observances, and other activities important to the patient. The profile should answer these questions: "What kind of person is this?" or "What is this person like?" "If I were around this person on an average day what might I learn about his or her style of interaction, inner self, soul?" The profile encourages interacting with the *patient as a person* rather than as an object. Asking the questions directed at "profiling" builds the caregiver-patient relationship. The profile may also include a statement as to the reliability of the information given by the patient.

Present illness or major active problem(s) (MAP) is a description of the nature and sequence of the patient's symptomatology as synthesized from the interview(s), old records, and referral data (including history, physical exam, lab work, X-ray). If there is more than one MAP, number and describe them separately unless they are very closely related.

Past illnesses and surgery, lists in varying detail important illnesses and surgeries from the past.

Review of systems is a detailed compendium of data from each organ system elicited through a series of standard, focused (mostly short-answer) questions

Social history, personal history, and family history contain information about the patient's life and family.

Physical exam (PE) records the findings on the physical exam, emphasizing those that supplement and clarify the interview and history data—the patient's story.

Diagnostic tests include the basic lab data (e.g., X-rays) for this encounter.[2]

Table 9.1 Sources of Data and Their Organization in the Chart

Organization of Database in Chart	Sources of Data						
	Interviews			Old Records Referral Data Phone	Exams		Routine Lab X-rays
	Patient		Family and Friends				
	Narrative	Focused			PE	MSE[a]	
Presenting circumstances or chief complaint	M	M	P	P			
Patient profile	M		M	P	P	P	
Major active problems or present illness	M	M or D	P	M or P	M	P	P or D
Past illnesses and surgery	M	M	P	M	M	P	P or D
Review of systems	P	M	P	P	P	P	
Personal and social history	M	M	M or P		P		
Family history	P	M	M	L	L		
Risk factors	M	M	P	P	P	P	D

NOTE: M = major contributor; D = definite contributor; L = lesser contributor; P = possible contributor.
a. Mental status exam.

Importance and Strategies of the Initial Contact

The patient comes to the physician with a characteristic mixture of hope and fear. He hopes that the physician will be able to discover the cause of his discomfort and take appropriate steps to set things right. At the same time he fears that the physician may not be able to help him and, in some instances, that help is not possible. (Enelow & Swisher, 1972, p. 29)

Your initial contact with a patient can set the tone for the relationship. Although you can overcome bad starts, it is much easier to start well. For newly admitted patients, you will be the first student and sometimes the first care-giver to see them. Other patients, previously assigned to your student prede-cessors, will also be new to you. *Honoring the patient* (Chapter 7) must *begin the first time you meet him or her.*

The goals of the first and subsequent early meetings are these:

- *To learn about your patient as a person who is ill or injured. No one is a disease or injury attached to a body.* There is no such thing as "just another angina." A patient with multiple sclerosis said, "I'm not a cripple; I'm a person with MS." In a sense, any clinical condition in the abstract is a fiction. Only when embodied is it real, and *every* embodiment is unique.

- *Establish rapport and trust.* If you're already busy and the situation is not acute, go to the patient's room soon after admission, introduce yourself, and establish a time for a longer visit.

- *Discuss mutual expectations and responsibilities.* If there is not enough time on the initial encounter, be sure to do it later; it is extremely important.

- *Convey an attitude of respectful caring.* By doing the first four of the following, substantial progress toward these stated goals can be made in only a few minutes. If you are comfortable, do the last one also. Appear unhurried!

  - **Address the patient as Mrs., Ms., Mr., or when appropriate, as "Doctor" or "Reverend" until he or she suggests use of his or her first name. Don't use nicknames.**

  - Ascertain or convey awareness of the patient's presenting circumstance.

  - Determine if the patient is feeling ill, in pain, feverish, nauseated, short of breath, or unexpectedly lethargic.

  - Tell the patient you are part of the patient care team, his or her advocate and in-terpreter of medical jargon.

  - If the patient appears depressed, anxious, fearful, or agitated, acknowledge your awareness of this and perhaps say, "It's understandable that you feel . . . and we will do our best to help you." Acknowledge pain and other ways in which he or she may be suffering.

In every initial contact, you will be memorable and impor-tant to the patient.

Collecting Data:
Overview and General Comments

In the interest of holistic, person-centered appraisal, we suggest reviewing Chapter 7 on honoring the patient. Also, remember the following: **When talking to the patient, make good eye contact.** This single behavior will do more than any other to establish and maintain trust and rapport.

The length of the interview varies, depending on circumstances, your pressures, and the complexity of the patient's problems. A brand-new hospitalization may require a lengthy initial appraisal. A new problem in an established patient requires more time than most routine follow-up visits. Emergency interviews may be quite brief or impossible.

There is a variable time course for clinical decision making. In an emergency, critical information must be obtained quickly. In other situations, however, all of the essential history may not emerge during one interview—even a long one. Lab data and physical findings change with time. Therefore, many problem solutions and diagnoses evolve over days or weeks.

On an outpatient clerkship, you will do complete appraisals on some new patients. Patients new to you but not to the clinic will have already had a complete appraisal. However, your teachers may tell you to do a new appraisal anyway because the patient is particularly instructive, in need of review, or because the database is incomplete.

Emergencies, language barriers, or a large new patient load may limit the comprehensiveness of initial appraisals. Agree with your clerkship director on a less exhaustive protocol for such difficult periods.

The following story shows how unexpected and important data can emerge from a complete appraisal:

> A student admitted a 45-year-old African American female with extensive edema and severe anemia. She had five prior admissions for renal failure that was mitigated by fluid management and peritoneal dialysis. She was barely able to continue work over the six months prior to admission. For financial/insurance reasons, she was not eligible for chronic dialysis. Taking a long shot, the student asked if she had a twin. She did—*an identical twin*—the perfect donor for a renal transplant. Why had she not been offered this alternative before? Careful examination of the records for all six of her admissions, including 18 H&Ps (a student, intern, and resident on each admission), disclosed that she had never been asked whether she had a twin!

The Interview and Patient Narrative

Patient Narrative

Despite sophisticated diagnostic techniques, the interview remains our single most powerful tool, giving rise to the patient's narrative and other valuable history. It may reveal how the patient and his or her family react to illness and (with the mental status exam) give clues to emotional and psychiatric disorders. The emergence (75%), accuracy, and completeness of diagnoses (assessments) are highly dependent on the interview (i.e., 75% of the patient's diagnoses or problems emerge during the interview; the accuracy and completeness of them often requires the PE and diagnostic tests and procedures) (Burack & Carpenter, 1983; Peterson, Holbrook, Von Hales, et al., 1992). Any gaps or deficiencies in data may be remedied by focused questioning later.

Of utmost importance, the interview is a foundation of the doctor-patient relationship. Sadly, many physicians, some in practice a long time, interview poorly. It is a privileged luxury of students to spend more time with patients than anyone else. You can really listen to their story and come to know them as people.

Basic Rules of Interviewing

Be as pleasant as possible. Learn to be genuinely genial even when pressured. If a patient is obtuse, chatty, or responds to your questions at great (and irrelevant) length, say, "I need to learn about you and your illness, but my time is limited. Please help me by being more brief."

Interview extremely ill, suffering, or moribund persons as briefly as possible. Extreme pain, shortness of breath, and frequent vomiting are all good reasons to limit your interview to obtaining essential data.

Use alternative sources of information when necessary or helpful. If the patient has been seen in this setting before, get the old charts and look for relevant lab reports, X-rays, and physical findings. For example, a patient with recurrent heart failure now has 3+ pretibial edema, rales at the right base, and atrial fibrillation. Were those findings present on the previous admission two months ago?

In situations (e.g., coma) in which the patient cannot communicate, family members, friends, and the old chart can be of great help. If a patient became unconscious at work, a phone call may tell you whether unconsciousness was sudden or gradual, if the patient complained of a headache beforehand, and other useful information. Sometimes a passerby will witness a medical or traumatic emergency and give helpful information.

The interview can be done in segments. If your write-up is already in the chart, you can make additions (in the progress notes) under the title, "Addition to Database." Some units may have a different way of charting this. Ask about it.

Ensure a minimum of interruptions. For an inpatient, pull curtains around the bed and close the door.

Skills of Interviewing[3]

Introduce yourself to the patient as a medical student. Review "Importance and Strategies of the Initial Contact" (above). Do not forget to maintain good eye contact. For effective interviewing, observe the following guidelines as consistently as possible.

Be aware of your position relative to the patient. When the patient is recumbent in bed or on an exam table, you should sit, not stand. Choose the side of the bed most comfortable for the patient, usually the side least encumbered with tubes, lines, and other equipment.

For ambulatory patients, sit within two to four feet of them, without a desk or other barrier between you. If the patient's condition permits, have him or her sit in a chair rather than sit or lie on the exam table.

Use open-ended inquiry to facilitate the emergence of narrative themes. Although some patients do not respond to even the most expert open-ended facilitation, most will relate the essence of their narrative in response to a few open-ended questions. "Say only enough to keep him going" (Bird, 1955, p. 11). The optimal questions will vary with the patient's personality and communication style, the nature of his or her problem(s), and time available. Begin with, "Tell me what's been happening," or "Tell me about this illness."

Open-ended questions often unearth unexpected clues about the disorder and/or the patient's personality: "When I'm having the pain, I get really cranky." "My wife got irritated because I hadn't helped with the dishes." "Eating gives me cramps, and then I have another bowel movement."

Ethan, 27, was admitted for treatment of tenacious and destructive substance abuse by order of the criminal justice system following two arrests for DUI. Dr. Barnes, an addiction specialist, knew the power of denial and the difficulty in establishing a trusting relationship with addicts. "Tell me what has been going on for you," she asked. The patient, clearly surprised by the question, gave an answer in which he revealed major painful emotional episodes from childhood and an essentially fatherless existence. He used drugs as anesthesia for the resultant emotional pain and suffering. Later, Dr. Barnes asked, "How do you see your life going from here?" This question elicited confusion, tears, and a deeply poignant "God, I don't know!"

If Dr. Barnes had asked, "How long have you had this problem?" "How much have you been drinking lately?" "When did you start using crack?" and continued with more focused questions, it is doubtful that she would have gained the same quality of information. Her respectful, open-ended questions honored the patient's sensitivities, intelligence, and autonomy. **Help the patient tell his or her own story.** Where possible avoid "yes," "no" questions. "How is your love life?" is better than, "Is your sex life good?" Important facts (frequency of the pain; is it dull, sharp; where exactly is it . . .) that do not emerge can be asked for later.

However, some patients respond too lavishly to open-ended questions. To the invitation, "tell me about your problem," you may receive a 10-minute (plus!), nonstop, detailed account of symptoms embellished with sidebars. It is too fast and jumbled to adequately comprehend. When this occurs, you must stop the patient, explain that this visit is time limited and that certain information has priority. You can then redirect the interview as needed.

Some clerkship guides suggest ways to keep the patient "on track" (i.e., "keep their responses brief") as you take their history. There are times (previous paragraph) when this is appropriate, but more often, it interferes with the emergence of valuable information. Remember you have more time to spend with patients than others on the team, and patience may open further windows on their personhood.

Be alert for signs of fear, anxiety, anger, sadness, and other signal emotions. A lot is learned from visual cues. Tune in to nervous facial expressions and body language: poor eye contact, the tapping foot, wringing hands, early tears, restlessness or its contrast, restricted body movement. The withdrawn or seductive patient may be hiding feelings.

When you suspect hidden emotion, it may be helpful to facilitate its expression: "You seem sad." "You look like you're about to cry." "It feels to me like you are angry." Overt expression of important feelings should be acknowledged and validated: "I can understand why you are sad." "Your anger feels appropriate to me." "That must, indeed, have been a joyful event."

If the patient is receptive, explore his or her spiritual and religious life during the interview. This is a rarely emphasized aspect of the appraisal that often reveals resources to support and supplement healing. Queries to initiate such a discussion are found in Chapter 19.

Explore the nature and degree of your patient's suffering (see Chapter 16). This issue is so neglected by medical educators that it might be called the *absent* curriculum.

Consciously differentiate the content and process of the interview. *Content* is what the patient reports to you. *Process* is what you learn about the patient from observation and his or her style of interaction. For anyone, self-reporting can be limited or altered by emotions and secrecy. Clues are often visible in the patient's behavior, facial expressions, body language, and speech patterns. The interview is an interpersonal experience. It reveals a lot about the patient's interpersonal style when under stress. **Pay close attention to appearance and nonverbal behavior.** Pain, shortness of breath, and sweating may be evident. Usually an acknowledgment of evident tension will be helpful.

Process data also includes your reactions, feelings, and behavior and their effect on the patient and the interview. Something the patient says may arouse your own feelings. At times, it is helpful to acknowledge that. For example, following an account of the patient's being abused, "I wonder if you're as angry about that as I am?" You may disregard important parts of the patient's narrative because it is uncomfortable for you. Your "stuff" can interfere with assessment and treatment of patients.

As one student interviewed a 48-year-old male with pneumonia, the patient became more relaxed and talkative. Asked about his family, the patient said, "My wife and I argue about her incessant nagging. She's on me all the time for pretty trivial stuff—like where I put my keys down when I come home." The student asked, "How old is your wife?" Then, "Does she have a job?" He went on to the system review and never came back to the discord. The resident explored the issue at length and included "Wife's Nagging" on the patient's master problem list. The resident also explored the student's diffidence. Apparently the student's parents had a similar dynamic for years, and six months earlier, had gotten a divorce. The student still harbored pain and anger. *He did not even remember the patient mentioning his wife's nagging!*

Use silence to help the patient respond. If a patient responds to your open-ended questions reluctantly or not at all or seems on the verge of expressing emotion, silence can be catalytic. Expectant silence also helps when the patient pauses to remember certain details or find the right words. He or she may say, "Let's see if I can be clearer." Or "Darn, I can't remember." However, the patient must see you as receptive. *Your demeanor needs to say, "I'm here, I am interested in what you are saying, take your time."* Don't look at the chart, stare vacantly across the room, sigh deeply, speak to another patient, or appear restless. Many physicians and students are uncomfortable with silence. If you are one of them, 30 seconds feels like a millennium. You must resist the urge to abort a pregnant pause.

Some patients (often teenagers) are particularly uncomfortable with silence. Be alert to this possibility and adjust accordingly.

Encourage further talk from the patient. Nodding, repeating the patient's last few words, a puzzled look or, "I don't understand," are ways of encouraging the temporarily "stuck" person to continue. Another important strategy is to return, at an appropriate lull, to a topic covered earlier but not completed. "You mentioned that your chest pain might be related in some way to your mother's visits. Please say more about that."

Use confrontation wisely. This is a valuable interviewing tool that is often misused. **Watch good interviewers. Ask how they handle certain situations.** If some of the patient's answers seem unlikely or untrue, do not confront him or her until there is confirmation—and definitely not the first time you are with the patient. The interview must not feel like the "first degree."

For confrontations intended to encourage lifestyle changes (such as smoking cessation) or acceptance of new treatment, the cardinal rule is to use data from inarguable sources: excerpts from the patient's own interview, physical findings ("I find many wheezes in your lungs"), lab work, X-ray and other test reports, remarks made by family or friends in the patient's presence, judicial penalties (DUI's). Reiterate diagnoses and "hard data" from the chart. For a cardiac patient, you might read the conclusions in a recent emergency room report. For an active alcoholic, list all previous treatment programs, the physical findings and lab data that support bodily damage (such as telangiectases, breast enlargement, elevated liver function tests) and any adverse consequences—family, workplace, social, financial—from alcohol. These data will be far more persuasive than your opinion or judgment. Give opinions if asked for, but as a motivating force, they are usually less helpful than we think.

When patients contradict themselves, consider confrontation: "Mr. Scharf, when I asked how you and your son get along you answered 'OK.' Since that point in our conversation, you have mentioned three recent loud arguments with him. What about that?"

If the patient's verbal report and nonverbal behavior are discrepant, it may also be worth confronting. He may report, "I am not a nervous person," but for 15 minutes he has tapped his foot and repeatedly shifted position. "What's happening Mr. Olivier? You seem nervous."

Use questions wisely. Focused questions represent the interviewing behavior most likely to produce biased information. As previously stated, open-ended questions facilitate emergence of the patient narrative. A number of short-answer questions (e.g., "Is the chest pain brought on by exertion?") will be necessary to fill out the database. **Before beginning focused questioning, alert the patient so he or she won't feel pigeonholed or objectified.**

Questions implying judgment, criticism, or suggested behavior are undesirable. They imply that he or she *should* be doing something. For example, "Tell me about your smoking" is better than, "You mean you haven't cut down on your smoking?" Questions free of judgment produce more truthful answers.

"Why?" questions are usually not helpful—"Why do you smoke (or drink) so much?" "Why" questions make people defensive and demand a reply. The answer is usually complex (genetics, socialization, present circumstances), and the response may be simplistic. "Why" questions also deflect or diminish the expression of feelings. A patient on the verge of tears can intellectualize on a why question, thereby screening out an important display of emotion.

Provide support and reassurance. Last, but far from least, the interview provides opportunities to give support and reassurance. Sincere support builds trust that encourages further productive exchange. "Support . . . communicates the interviewer's interest in, liking for, or understanding of the patient or promotes a feeling of security in the relationship" (Enelow & Swisher, 1972, p. 48). A sympathetic nod or brief statements such as, "I hear you," or "That must have been upsetting," are very supportive. Another helpful strategy is to briefly summarize what the patient has just said in a way that conveys "sympathetic comprehension." *Support is especially important following display of strong feelings: weeping, fear, or anger.* A caution, however: Facile words are worse than none at all. Patients quickly detect remarks that are insincere, tinged with disapproval, or not backed by an honest desire to be helpful. They will seem manipulative.

Reassurance must have similar qualities. Some students and physicians tend to respond to a patient's need for hope by overstating positive findings or progress. Insofar as possible, base reassurances on sound evidence. Do not use clichés ("Everything is going to be fine,") when they're not appropriate. As with support, the attitudes underlying reassurance must be congruent. Dishonesty and subterfuge, even with fine motives, will be perceived by most patients.

Activity: Each day for a week, practice one or two of the interviewing skills just reviewed. Try them out on family members, partners, friends, and colleagues.

Physical Exam

The physical exam (PE) provides valuable information that cannot be obtained in other ways; it is a logical extension of the interview. In physical diagnosis, you have probably been *taught* what constitutes a good PE. Whether you have *learned* a proficient exam is another question.

The Interview as Entrée

Except in certain emergencies, the interview is an essential prerequisite to the exam—to enhance rapport, trust, and appropriate congeniality. *Done in isolation, the exam may be felt as an invasion of privacy, or worse, as an assault.* Also, your manner and talk during the physical exam and how you report your findings to the patient all influence your relationship with him.

Even in short outpatient follow-up visits, spend a few minutes interviewing the patient before checking physical findings. Given a patient with a kidney infection under treatment with antibiotics, start with an open-ended question such as, "How's it been going?" then proceed to more focused inquiry: "How often are you urinating?" "Any burning when you urinate?" "Any fever?" Such an approach will provide an entré to examine the patient's back for costovertebral angle tenderness, his abdomen for kidney enlargement and bladder tenderness, his face and ankles for edema, the rectum for prostate abnormalities, and to take his blood pressure.

Getting Help to Improve

Practice with supervision is the best way to become proficient. Ask a resident or an attending to observe you through at least one complete exam. When you do isolated exam procedures during rounds, ask your teacher(s) to critique your technique as well as your findings. When they suggest that you examine a certain patient's abdomen (heart, neck, etc.), ask them not to reveal the findings beforehand.

Try different techniques and question people using different techniques. Are there advantages over your way? For example, liver size can be assessed by percussion, palpation, and by placing your stethoscope over the liver as you scratch the right abdominal wall in ascending strokes. The auscultatory tone changes when you reach the liver edge. Ask different specialists to help you increase your PE skills in their specialty area.

Suggested Sequencing of the Physical Examination

The sequence for the PE shown in Table 9.2 is efficient, reduces errors and omissions, and requires minimum movement or changes in position for the patient. The suggested sequence, beginning with the patient's head, runs down the left-hand column of the table. Obviously, other basic sequences are possible. The important thing is that you use the same sequence most of the time. It may be desirable to modify your sequence to examine painful areas last—especially in children. Different sequences may be imperative in times of emergency or acute patient discomfort. However, all good sequences *flow*.

In each step of the PE, you will use one or (usually) more of the following modalities: *inspection, palpation, percussion, auscultation*. In most regions of the body, you will augment or enhance your exam by asking the patient to change position, breathe deeply, or move in certain ways, or by using an instrument such as a light, a speculum, a tongue blade, a reflex hammer, or the stethoscope (in fact, almost all your auscultation will be done with the stethoscope).

Table 9.2   Sequencing the Physical Exam

Body Region	Foci of Attention	Notes
Head	Cranium, scalp, ears, eyes (NS), nose, mouth (teeth, tongue, throat), facial movements and sensations (NS)	You can begin the neurological exam here: e.g., the pupillary responses and movements of the eye, facial movements, and facial sensations all assess various cranial nerves.
Neck	Cervical spine, veins, pulses, cervical nodes, thyroid	Assess range of motion of head and neck.
Axillae	Nodes, tenderness, sweating	So far everything can be done with the patient sitting or lying on his or her back.
Arms	Musculature, pulses, joints, reflexes, sensation (NS)	Check radial pulses with arms down, then raised in "hands-up" position.
Back	Thoracic and lumbosacral spine, skin of back (it may be the only time you'll see it), CVA[a] region	This may be the first time you have to change the patient's position.
Thorax	Thoracic cage, lungs, heart, breast (get special instruction in protocol and technique for breast exam)	Inspection/palpation is very important here, often neglected because of preoccupation with auscultation. Chest pain is often from the chest wall and may be referred from the abdomen.
Abdomen	Organ size, abnormal masses or pulsations, tenderness, bowel sounds, fluid, abd. reflexes (NS)	Do exam with patient on back, soles of feet on table, knees bent up to relax abdominal wall.
Male genitalia	Penis, testicles, check for hernia cremasteric reflex (NS)	If uncircumcised, have patient draw foreskin back.
Legs	Musculature, veins, pulses, joints, reflexes, sensation (NS)	Check for edema and calf tenderness.
Anus/rectum	Perianal area, prostate (in males), masses, tenderness	Position patient on side, knees drawn up. Look for hemorrhoids. **Observe protocol re chaperone.**
Neurological exam	**Seek advice on how extensive a neurological exam to do on any given patient.** At this point, what you do depends on what you have done along the way (e.g., DTRs,[b] pupillary responses and EOM,[c] abdominal and cremasteric reflexes).	You may prefer to do all the neurological exam at once. **Remember that most neurological information comes from the face, eyes, legs, and arms.**
Genitalia/ pelvic (women)	Vulva, clitoris, labia, vagina, cervix, body of uterus, tubes, ovaries	**Observe protocol re chaperone.** A female nurse can act as chaperone and help with Pap smears and other tests.

a. Costovertebral angle.
b. Deep tendon reflexes.
c. Extraocular movement.

Remember also that you have the option of assessing the patient's neurological status as you proceed through the various body regions (places marked in
Table 9.2 with NS) or of doing all the neurological testing together. **Inspect
(and when indicated, palpate) the skin at any/all stages of the exam. Do not
forget it.**

Talking to the Patient During the Exam

Talk with the patient during the exam. Rapport builds when you inform the
patient of your next move and about your findings as you proceed. It is an ideal
time to do the system review and elicit further details about the past or present
history. Silence during the exam (except when using the stethoscope) may be
ominous to the patient. Examining a particular area as you question about it
may stimulate the patient to recall certain past events—forgotten until now. To
minimize anxiety, ask the first question for each organ system ("Any problems
in the past with your bladder or kidneys?") *before* you begin to examine the
corresponding parts of the body.

Respect the Patient's Feelings

In our society there are few (legal!) professional situations in which one person has the expectation and privilege of viewing and touching another who is
disrobed. Like parts of the interview, this intimacy is an integral part of the
doctor-patient relationship. It is necessary and expected. Nevertheless, it creates anxiety for the patient. "The fully clothed physician must always be aware
of the . . . shame, embarrassment, and feelings of inferiority that his unclothed
patient may experience." Examinations of the breasts, vagina, external genitalia, and rectum, can be particularly susceptible to misinterpretation if not done
in a professional manner. Proper draping, courtesy, and not lingering "over
these emotion-laden areas" are usually sufficient to lessen the patient's discomfort (Enelow & Swisher, 1972, p. 123). At times, however, evidence of increasing anxiety as the exam proceeds (perhaps anticipating your exam of the
"emotion-laden areas," perhaps as the examiner nears the part of the body that
is afflicted), requires sensitive exploration: "I notice that you seem to feel embarrassed. How can I help with that?" then silence. Or "I see the exam is difficult for you; it might help to discuss that." In the event of affliction-focused
anxiety, it is often enough to say, "It feels to me like you might be worried about
what I might find in your stomach (heart, uterus) . . ."

Student Anxieties

You may feel anxious about doing physical exams because of the intimacy involved. Even after considerable experience, particular situations may provoke anxiety (such as a severely injured patient or a seductive one). When aware of this, try not to telegraph your anxiety by hurrying—particularly over the emotionally charged areas. Ask about policies on the service with respect to chaperones. As a general rule, a chaperone should be present when the breasts, heart, external genitalia, rectum, and pelvis of a woman are examined and for exam of the rectum and external genitalia in a man. If a patient is titillated by an examiner, it is appropriate to terminate the exam or cover the genitalia and move on to a less sensitive area (e.g., extremities, neurological examination). Any patient may refuse all or certain parts of the exam. In these circumstances, talk to your attending or clerkship coordinator. Reassignment of the patient may be necessary at times. Talk about your anxieties to trusted colleagues, a mentor, and/or your support group.

While you're still inexperienced, it is common and highly understandable to be anxious about your proficiency. One student said, "Sometimes I wonder 'how long should I listen to this guy's heart?' I really don't know what I'm hearing and if I listen too long, he'll know I don't know what I'm doing, or worse yet, he might start worrying that I've found something wrong" (Coombs, 1998, p. 104). Practice and good supervision are the answer to this one!

Touching

Appropriate touch can strengthen your relationship with patients. Two suggestions may help. First, touch with confidence. You can do this even though you may be anxious because this is your first PE or because you find the patient particularly attractive. Affirm silently, "My touch will be confident and reassuring, not unhelpful or confusing in any way." Second, with both sexes, it is courteous and respectful to cover the patient, exposing only those areas under examination.

Unfacilitated Observation

This is an important aspect of the physical exam. It is taught poorly, if at all. A lot of information is available through your eyes and ears alone without using hands, instruments, or giving instructions. Examples include the following: the characteristic (and different) deformities of degenerative arthritis and rheumatoid arthritis in the fingers, the excessive perspiration of anxiety and hyperthyroidism, the fine tremor and protuberant eyes also seen in hyperthyroidism, the channeled nails of iron deficiency, poor dental hygiene, various abnormalities suggesting neurological problems, the nicotine-stained fingers of the inveterate smoker, and the barrel chest of advanced emphysema. When patients are on the exam table before the examiner enters the room, and after he or she leaves, we may forfeit the opportunity to watch the patient walk and dress, two activities that can provide a lot of "unfacilitated" data.

Surface Anatomy

Most internal organs occupy a characteristic place beneath the surface of the body (see Figure 9.1), and pain from a given organ often presents in the same area.

With knowledge of surface anatomy, you can better interpret your exam findings and assess possible organ damage from stabbings, other penetrating wounds, or trauma. It will also help to differentiate certain problems. For example, a patient complains of left anterior chest pain. From the interview, you may or may not already know the most likely explanations for it. Assuming that you do not yet have a cause, surface anatomy tells you that the pain might be from the chest wall, the pleura, the heart, the mediastinum (containing the esophagus, aorta, great veins, and lymph nodes), or from a distended splenic flexure of the colon. It might be referred from the spine or spinal nerve roots. As you examine the chest, heart, lungs, spine, and abdomen, you focus on differentiating these possibilities. Is there tenderness of the chest wall, a gallop rhythm, a pleural friction rub, decreased or absent breath sounds, changes in sensory perception, or a pocket of air in the splenic flexure? Similar analysis and differentiation in other parts of the body can be extremely helpful.

Recording the Appraisal

Table 9.1 and Box 9.1 give a suggested format for recording your appraisal (which will be called "your H&P" by most teachers). Your service may require a different format. The patient profile in some coherent, recognizable form may not be part of their format. If not, add it to the proscribed format using the heading "Patient Profile."

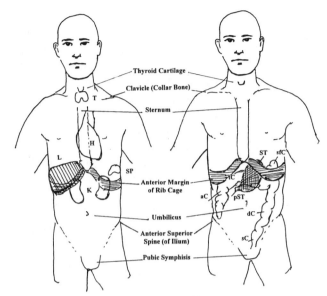

Figure 9.1. Surface Anatomy

In somewhat idealized fashion this figure shows the approximate surface representation of the major organs on the anterior surface of the body. The externally visible or palpable body landmarks are indicated by labels connected to the landmark by solid lines. The organs themselves are labeled within the figures using the following abbreviations:

T	= thyroid gland	H	= heart and aortic arch	SP	= spleen	
L	= liver	K	= kidneys	ST	= stomach	
				pST	= pylorus	
sfC	= splenic flexure of colon			aC	= ascending colon	
tC	= transverse colon	dC	= descending colon	sC	= sigmoid colon	

In the authors' experience the frontal representation of a *normal heart* often extends 1-3 cm further to the left in the patient than shown and sometimes 2-4 cm further downward toward the abdomen as well. The *lungs,* which are not labeled, fill all of the thoracic cavity not occupied by heart or mediastinum (most of the latter lies directly behind the sternum). Since the diaphragm is higher in the front than at the back, the lungs extend down as far as the 11th or 12th thoracic vertebra in the back.

Note that the *normal liver and spleen* are protected by the rib cage. They cannot be felt during examination of the abdomen unless they are enlarged or the diaphragm is depressed (as in severe emphysema). Further, with respect to the liver and not shown here, is that part of the L. lobe, in many normal people, extends to the left (patient's) of the mid-line. It will be tucked up under the diaphragm and may be behind the rib margin so it is seldom (unless enlarged) felt.

The *stomach* varies greatly in size depending on its fullness.

The *kidneys* are located far posteriorly. In a thin person they can sometimes be felt by deep palpation of the abdomen in the region between the umbilicus and the lower margins of the rib cage anteriorly. Posteriorly they lie along either side of the spine between about T-12 and L-2.

The *abdominal aorta* (not shown) also lies far posteriorly against the left side of spine. If the abdomen is soft, aortic pulsations can usually be felt on deep palpation above the umbilicus just to the left (patient's) of midline.

Notes

1. The nomenclature and system we have used so far, prefer, and will continue to use in this book is *problem oriented*. Your institution may not use problem-oriented charting, in which case the assessment section will probably not appear as such. Instead, there will be *diagnosis(es)* or *impression(s)*. There will probably be one *plan* that encompasses all of the entities mentioned in the list of diagnoses. Many places use a system that is a mixture of the older convention and the problem-oriented method.

2. Each service requires initial lab data that are routinely obtained on every patient. The exact tests performed may differ from specialty to specialty but also between two clerkships of the same specialty.

3. We are indebted to the authors of *Interviewing and Patient Care* (Enelow, Forde, & Brummel-Smith, 1996; Enelow & Swisher, 1972) for liberal use of their organizational patterns and thinking on the interviewing process. There are many instances in which we have, with their permission, paraphrased their work.

10 Rounds and Teamwork

Musical rounds sound wonderful when the groups sing well and synchronize properly; otherwise they are dysphonic. Medical rounds are like that too!

In older hospitals, beds were situated around the periphery of a large room. "Medical rounds" classically referred to the moving discussion of doctors and nurses from bedside to bedside. Today (in both inpatient and outpatient settings) we use *rounds* to mean any series of sequential discussions about patients by the professionals responsible for them. Nowadays, all rounds are not held at the bedside or in the outpatient examining room. Many are in the doctors' teaching area or a conference room. Sadly, some patients discussed on rounds are not actually seen by the group.

There are (a) work rounds with house staff, (b) attending rounds, (c) your own private rounds, (d) chart rounds, (e) subspecialty or consultant rounds, and (f) morning report (see Table 10.1). As students, you will participate with house staff and/or attending physicians in most of these. Although some rounds are primarily for one or the other, patient care and teaching meet in rounds (Table 10.1).

To be effective, rounds require teamwork. There is almost always a leader and a pecking order. The hierarchy may be rigidly maintained (people are always questioned in the same order, titles are carefully used, etc.) or quite democratic. Regardless, the medical student is invariably low on the totem pole.

Work Rounds With House Staff

Work rounds are essential for good patient care. When possible, see your assigned patients beforehand and *be prepared with the latest lab results, vital*

Table 10.1 Types of Rounds

Types of Rounds	Participants	Primary Purpose	Work Done
Attending	Attendings, house staff, students, nurses(s)	Review and coordinate patient care; update diagnosis & management; discuss fine points as time permits	Present new findings; talk with patient; examine as necessary; assess progress; write new orders; DC[a] those no longer needed
Work	House staff, students, head nurse	Review present status & orders; DC as necessary; check, revise management as indicated	Review cardex; status reports from nurses, PGY, or student; update lab and X-ray
Subspecialty or consulting	Subspecialty attending, fellow or resident, student as possible	Review and coordinate diagnosis and care of subspecialty-focused problems	Discuss patient problems with subspecialty focus; do or schedule special diagnostic procedures
Private	Student (and PGY)	Answer patient questions; update patient information regarding tests & changes; develop relationship	Talk with patient; repeat pertinent exam items; provide sincere reassurance as possible
Chart	Single person or group of 2-5 (as on work rounds)	See that charts are in order & up to date	Go through charts systematically; write orders/make entries to fill gaps
Morning report	Chief of Service or surrogate, residents, students sometimes	Highlights of previous day; sketch notable new admissions	Occasional decisions made about management

a. Discontinue.

signs, symptomatology, and physical findings (e.g., daily weights on the person with congestive heart failure, blood sugars on diabetics). Check with the team that took night call for any new information.

A few purists believe students should commit everything to memory. We advocate the use of a small notebook or handheld computer in which you can jot the latest data and reminders. Sir William Osler wrote, "You can do nothing as a student in practice without [note taking]. Carry a small notebook . . . and never ask a new patient a question without notebook and pencil in hand" (Osler, 1995, p. 32).

Although a presentation from memory will impress your faculty, on work rounds it is usually acceptable to use the chart. However, don't waste time leafing through it; know where the data you need can be found. To begin discussion on one of your ongoing patients, present a *brief* summary and update. Here's an example:

> "This is the third hospital day for Mr. Dubois, who is 51. He was admitted with shortness of breath and found to have pneumonia. He is a longtime two-pack-a-day smoker. On amoxicillin and fluids, he is afebrile, breathing 16 times per minute, and at 6 a.m. his blood gases were normal. Repeat chest film and bronchoscopy have been ordered. No complications have occurred."

The time spent with each patient will vary. If the patient's status is unstable, it may be important to ask several questions or check certain physical findings. It is best, however, not to get into a prolonged conversation with him or her on work rounds. Wait until you can come back and spend solo time. Your patients will appreciate this, and it will strengthen your relationship with them. Perceptive house staff will encourage this strategy. "Your medical student or I will be back later to talk more with you." **Before leaving each patient, make notes on new tasks expected of you—orders to be written and data to be checked.**

Attending Rounds

On most clerkships, students make attending rounds with the house staff, but on some, they make rounds separately. Then the attending can direct all questions and instruction—such as improving physical examination skills—to the students.

Some attendings discuss only one or two patients; others want to know the status of every patient and have input on every management decision. Hopefully, you will be expected to present the initial appraisal (Chapter 9) on any of your patients the attending has not seen. Your offering should be concise and organized and should convey enough information for the attending to formulate a list of the most important problems. Don't go on and on just to be thorough. Present your patient by beginning with a problem list that discriminates between old and currently active problems. If the problem that led to the present encounter is a new one, you might omit it. Then, proceed with a short narrative from which the new problem can be identified and named. Here's an example:

This 46-year-old married, Asian male enters with "heavy" chest pain. His known problems include hypertension, posttraumatic ACL repair, and psoriasis. The chest pain began four hours prior to admission, in the mid-anterior chest, accompanied by sweating, nausea, and some shortness of breath. There was no cough, calf pain, or history of trauma to the chest. He had not done any weight lifting for several days before admission. He denies fever, palpitations, or previous episodes of this kind. In the emergency room, he was anxious, sweating, and breathing at 20 X a minute. Temp 99.8, pulse 80 with 4 to 6 premature contractions per minute and occasional 3- to 5-second runs of a more rapid rate. Chest was clear to P and A; he was not coughing; there was no ankle or leg edema; the calves were soft and nontender; no cyanosis. EKG suggested acute myocardial injury. He was admitted stat via stretcher with the new problem of myocardial ischemia and impending infarction.

Activity: With the patient's permission, record one of your bedside presentations on audiotape. Listening to it later can be invaluable for self-assessment and improvement of your "on stage" time.

Other Types of Rounds

Table 10.1 stipulates the participants, primary purpose, and work of six types of rounds, two of which have already been discussed. Check with your clerkship director, resident, or attending to learn which ones you will need to attend and which may be optional.

Problems With Rounds

Stressful presentations, a lethargic pace, personal fatigue (it may be hard to stay awake!), power struggles, and subtle put-downs can make rounds difficult. Outright humiliation is rare, but it may occur and is a matter to report to the clerkship director or an ombudsman.

1. *Gamesmanship* on rounds is not uncommon. The "pearl game" is popular. In life, pearls are nice but not essential. The same is true of teaching pearls. They are fun and sometimes instructive but often have little relevance to the pathophysiology or management of the problem at hand. An attending who drops a lot of pearls may preen his or her ego to the detriment of the teaching process. One attending asked a student the causes of "crenated red blood cells" on the peripheral blood smear. The student did well by mentioning technically poor blood smear, sickle cell anemia, and renal failure. The attending coaxed her on, but the student drew a blank. "Well," said the attending, "such cells are seen in a-beta-lipoproteinemia." At that time, less than 20 cases had been identified in the world. To divert the inveterate pearl dropper, redirect the learning process to the diagnostic and treatment issues of the patient under discussion.

2. Another more subtle game is *one-upmanship*. A resident, threatened by a knowledgeable student, asks an obscure question or recalls a noteworthy therapeutic victory involving a patient the student has never seen. This can distract the attending from the current case and from the student who "knows more."

3. During rounds a patient is disregarded or devalued when the bedside discussion becomes a debate about the problem in general or discussion of another patient with a similar problem. While helpful to learners, the patient may feel disregarded.

4. Power struggles or a particularly needy or defensive teacher can diminish the quality of rounds. If you suspect this, here are some suggestions:

- Don't get involved in power struggles (especially on rounds) and controversy (veiled or open), such as "who heard the murmur first."
- Give credit where credit is due (if you know with assurance).
- Don't become defensive even in the face of criticism.
- Take Osler's advice and have "a clear knowledge of (your) relation to your fellow creatures and to the work of life" (Osler, 1932a, p. 6), and consequently, don't expect too much of others.
- Don't expect your house staff and attendings to know everything or to sparkle in the instructional role; then all the instruction you receive will be a gift.

5. Rounds deal with life, death, and quality of life. We are sometimes reluctant to end discussion of a patient within a specified period of time. The best "rounders" we have known, however, are able to do just that, either explicitly

("time's up for this patient") or simply by moving on when the time becomes excessive.

Improving Rounds

Rounds are extremely important: to the patients, to students and house staff as learners, and to the attending as a means to coordinate the team's work. It is worth stating your concern if they are not accomplishing those purposes. The better the teamwork, the more effective rounds become.

Students can improve the effectiveness of rounds with quality presentations and good questions. If you keep things *problem focused,* have *specific questions* you want answered (and your own tentative answers ready), and keep your presentations *concise and pertinent,* those parts of rounds related to your patients will go well. If rounds are not meeting your expectations, talk with the senior resident on the service. Make suggestions about improving rounds—especially ways in which students can help.

Teamwork

Good patient care requires teamwork, in the setting of rounds, in the practitioner's office, and in the marshaling and coordination of community resources (home nursing, nutritional expertise, special care placement). Even solo practitioners have a team—nurse(s), office assistants, and others in the community. During your first intensive clerkship experiences, it is wise to pay attention to teamwork—what makes good teamwork and what barriers stand in its way.

Activity: During orientation to a new clerkship, make a list of your tasks and responsibilities. Also list the many tasks and responsibilities carried out by the nurses, orderlies, and other people who work on the unit. Is there overlap, conflict, gaps?

Suggestions for Being a Good Team Member

Teamwork is a frequently used term. We all think we know what it means, and most of us believe we are good team players.

For a student clerk, being an effective team member requires the following:

1. Acknowledge deeply that you are part of the team, not just an observer or student.

2. Find out (by asking, listening, and observing) what is expected of you by the attendings, residents, and nurses. Expectations may include some or all of the following:

   - Promptly complete all assigned patient appraisals (histories and physicals), and get the write-up into the chart.

   - Attend all scheduled rounds and team meetings.

   - Prepare for rounds: know all the new lab and X-ray results on your patients; know how they are responding to treatment; be prepared to present this data; on complicated patients, a chart on the blackboard is very helpful.

   - At first, mostly listen unless asked. After the first week or two, begin to offer suggestions and ask questions.

   - Make lists of all assigned tasks unless only one is given and you can do it right away.

   - Complete all tasks. Warn the attending or resident ahead of time if you won't finish something important on time.

3. Carry out those expectations to the best of your abilities.

4. Improve cooperation with your fellow students:

   - When overburdened, ask for help from a fellow student or arrange with the attending to have the work shared with others.

   - If you can manage it, offer help to fellow students who fall behind.

5. Spend time with the ward clerk (see Chapter 4).

6. Treat all other caregivers, including lab personnel, ward clerks, and transporters, as people, not servants; some have served long and faithfully, some have great stories to tell, all can be of real help to you.

7. If another team member's communication with patients is rude, indifferent, or apathetic, counteract this by modeling consideration and interest. Even though you are a medical student, it can have a surprisingly good effect.

We suggest you review the suggestions made in Chapter 4 about working with nurses and other unit personnel.

Suggestions for Working With Consultants

- Make every effort to see your patient with the consultant.

- If the consultant visits while you are occupied, speak to him or her before or afterward if possible to clarify what you need from the consult. This may avoid an additional phone call or contact.

- Initial the consultant's note in the chart and add a short acknowledgment such as, "Thanks, we will do 1-3 in your suggested plan." This is good communication.

- Ask any questions or about special needs in the consult request or progress notes; they may clarify the consultant's recommendations or thinking.

Disagreements

If you disagree with the house staff or attending physician about a patient's management, you will learn something. Disagreements are usually settled by a short discussion. However, you may be more sensitive to issues around heroic care and prolonging life than the attending or house staff (Chapter 14). You may, for example, find yourself in disagreement about the use of extreme measures to prolong life when an alternative might be better for the patient and the family.

> Jerry, a third-year clerk on medicine, admitted a 95-year-old woman from a nursing home. She had been bedridden and completely disoriented for six months and comatose for 48 hours. Her appraisal indicated a recent stroke, severe renal failure, and pulmonary infiltrates suggesting pneumonia or pulmonary infarct. The house staff did not contact the family before plunging into a vigorous regimen that included brisk hydration and electrolyte regulation, antibiotics for a suspected pneumonia, peritoneal lavage, and nasogastric alimentation. The attending physician reviewed the case briefly on the second hospital day and, by default, essentially agreed with the treatment. With house staff approval, Jerry phoned the son and sought an ethics consult. It was then decided, with the son's urging and concurrence, to limit treatment to hydration only.

Socializing With House Staff and Other Unit Personnel

This is a tricky issue. For students and residents, the intensity and collegiality of working together can generate solid friendships. A few last for years. Group socializing in one's time off by and large seems harmless. There will, inevitably, be parties.

Romantic involvement between a resident, a nurse, or other unit personnel and a student assigned to the same service is not a good idea—particularly if it includes sex. Romantic feelings are not always easy to hide in the work environment. One couple was transparent to an astute patient who embarrassed the pair on rounds by asking how long they had been "going together." If two people already involved are thrown together on a clerkship, the situation is a little different, although this should also be avoided when possible.

The pitfalls of a sexual liaison, no matter how "casual," are clear. First, the power differential between student and teacher (even when age is similar) is tricky enough without the condiment of sex. Second, an affair can create favoritism and/or jealousy. In one instance, a student's two clerkship colleagues felt that he was shown favoritism in the evaluations as the result of his sexual involvement with their resident. This created animosity from other classmates during the rest of medical school.

11 Working With Family and Other Loved Ones

> The conduct of the family interview can be very gratifying if the clinician is aware that despite the sense of fear, hurt, and even despair that may often be found in families experiencing a serious health crisis, most families have deep resources to draw upon in helping one another.
>
> —*C. Worby (1972, p. 160)*

A professional consciousness that encompasses the family is an invaluable asset to most physicians. An occasional family or family member can be an aggravation or a "loose cannon," but much more frequently, they are a sterling asset—although the "mining" may be difficult. On most clerkships, students have limited contact with families. Some (family medicine, internal medicine, pediatrics) may assign a family therapist to work specifically with house staff and students. Even then, some residents and attendings will not value family work. Nevertheless, through experience, most astute practitioners learn to value and facilitate the important contribution that families can make in the care, healing, and education of patients. Some doctors become proficient at conducting the family interview—a valuable tool for meaningful interaction with families.

Indications for
Involvement With the Family

Caregivers may interact fruitfully with a patient's family under most circumstances. In the following situations, family contact is especially desirable. More than one of the following situations may be dealt with in the same encounter.

At the Time of Major Life Events. Your family medicine and/or primary care continuity clerkships provide many opportunities to do valuable work with families (premarital exams, birth control counseling, pregnancy, well-child visits, camp physicals, periodic adult health checkups—such as the pap and pelvic exams).

During an Acute or Chronic Illness. You can exchange information in one or both of two ways. In the first, the clinician needs more information about the patient and his illness. New information and insights from the family can illuminate a diagnostic problem or provide medical history data that the patient cannot remember or communicate (because of coma, stroke, poor memory, etc.). In the second, the clinician provides a progress report to the family, discusses management strategies, or both—such as changes in medication or other treatment. Such contacts range from brief ones conveying the results of a test to much longer meetings that cover the patient's condition in great detail. Family members may hold varied ideas about the patient's illness, the proposed management, or both. A group interview can help them to a common understanding. Information sessions may be simple in their dynamics or very stressful, as when delivering bad news to the family—the patient has inoperable cancer or the patient has died. Honesty and realism are essential.

To Learn About Patterns of Family Interaction and Communication, Normally and During Stress. You can also help the family understand such patterns. This can improve both communication and the patient's care at home. The family may also reveal interactive patterns that affect the illness ("Dad's blood sugars are much higher when we're all fussing at one another"). Sometimes uncovering such patterns is the only purpose of the interview.

The discharge interview may combine both exchange of information and a look at family dynamics.

Examples of the
Family Influencing Outcomes

• Your patient recovers from an acute illness with good functional outcomes. You expect him or her to go home and function well. However, if the impact of the illness on family patterns was not considered, there may be profound unfavorable consequences after discharge.

> A 41-year-old obese assembly line worker with hypertension entered the hospital in coma after a sudden massive headache. Subarachnoid hemorrhage was quickly diagnosed, and the neurosurgeons successfully clipped a leaking aneurysm. The patient was fully conscious in 18 hours and recovered completely save for some memory loss and slight right-sided weakness. At home, the patient's wife became oversolicitous and drastically altered the entire family's meals to ensure her husband's adherence to the recommended low-fat, reducing diet. She drove him to places within easy walking distance, and sex was suspended for fear that "something might happen." A year after discharge, he was not back at work.

An interview with the family prior to discharge might have improved the likelihood that the patient could resume a functionally optimal lifestyle.

In a dramatic portrayal of contrasts, two men in their early 50s, each married with three children, are admitted to the hospital within a few days of each other, both with myocardial infarction (MI). They do well in the hospital. One has a lengthy family interview that includes instruction and encouragement on a course of self-care at home. The other is given the same information quite rapidly on rounds the morning of discharge. The first man does well and is back to work and other normal activities within six weeks. The second patient is "taken over" by a caring but insecure and controlling wife. He feels infantilized until an astute family therapist in the follow-up clinic discerns what is happening and arranges three family sessions. The wife "gets" that her neediness impedes her spouse's return to a functional life. As an unexpected dividend, the children reveal their fears that "Dad won't be able to go camping or play ball again."

• You think you have explained things lucidly to a patient's family only to find that they appear not to have heard.

A widow in her early 60s, admitted for a compound fracture of the hip, is found to also have adult-onset diabetes. It is easily controlled on caloric restriction. She is losing weight and has no sugar in her urine at the time of discharge. She lives with her son, his wife, and two young children—who continue to eat as they always have, consuming a lot of fatty food and "free" sugar. The patient's weight loss stops, and her next fasting blood sugar is 280 mg/100 ml (normal 60-120). Two family interviews are required to regain the lost ground.

• Despite assertions to the family that their husband and dad has a significant drinking problem, you find that your explanations were only partly heard, significantly misinterpreted, or denied.

An alcoholic man enters the hospital with acute pancreatitis. He has an enlarged liver, elevated liver function tests, and quadriceps atrophy. He gives a clear history of prolonged, heavy alcohol use and abuse. A family interview prior to discharge uncovers enabling behavior in the family, particularly in response to the patient's requests for alcohol. On the patient's return home, he continues to drink excessively. The wife continues to excuse his drinking, and his two adolescent sons control the household with their acting out. Two weeks after discharge, a family interview confirms that the family still has not accepted alcohol dependence as the basic problem to which the patient's pancreatitis, liver disease, and muscle atrophy are secondary.

How Medical Students Can Interact Usefully With Families

Be alert for situations that could profit from closer or more intense involvement of family. If you're not sure, ask your resident or attending. With proper supervision, you can do some things alone or organize family sessions to be led by the resident, the attending, or a family therapist. Here are some suggestions:

• If you need further information about the patient, look on the registration sheet of the chart. Often, the "to be notified" person can supply the information you need by phone or guide you to someone who can.

- A family meeting will shift the focus of attention (temporarily) from the patient to the family. Clarify the goals of such a shift (to gather or give information, to get to know the family better in ways that will help the patient, to update the family) with the patient.

- When talking with a family member or group, particularly if you have not met them before, try the following:

  - Find a reasonably quiet place to meet. The patient's room works unless there are other patients there. Meeting in hallways and at the nurse's station is bad form.
  - If your time is limited, say so before you begin the meeting.
  - Decide with a clinician or family therapist about whether the patient should be present. Judge each instance separately.
  - Whatever the purpose of the meeting, assure the family that questions will be answered.
  - Be honest and forthright about what you know unless the patient has asked you to limit disclosure. The patient might, for example, want his or her HIV status or the full severity of the situation withheld. Conversely, sometimes the family receives "bad news" first and wants part or all of it to be withheld from the patient. At this point, you need help from your resident, attending, or a family therapist.
  - When one person in a family interview dominates the interaction, use judgment about whether to exert control or not. Sometimes, cultural differences determine that only the eldest male, for example, may speak for the family in public. It is essential to respect these cultural norms.

- The more family members present for an update, the less likely the problem of distortion later on. Ask two or more of them to respond to the query, "What have you heard me say?"

- When a prime purpose of the interview is to learn something about family dynamics, try the following:

  - Open with something such as, "Well, how have things been for all of you?"
  - Watch for group patterns of interaction, such as a conspiracy of silence, one or more persons repeatedly speaking for someone else, dominance by one person, "taking sides."
  - Look for the family "MO" in dealing with strong feelings—for example, free expression, stoic and/or closed affect, substitution of behaviors for one emotion

or another (nervous laughter for fear), denial, deflection of sincere feelings expressed by others.

   – Look for recurring patterns in the way that family members relate to one another.

Activity: During your next major specialty clerkship, keep a list of all contacts with family members and other loved ones. What was achieved during each contact? Would more have been accomplished had you conducted the session differently?

When to Call the Family Therapist

If house staff and attendings are not inclined to, or not skilled at, facilitating interaction with the family, ask approval to find a medical social worker (MSW), psychologist, or family therapist. In many settings, the MSW is skilled at working with families. Having located such a person, briefly present your case, ask advice, and encourage him or her to see your patient.

Later, as a practicing physician, you may want to handle most "family matters" yourself. Here are some situations in which, as a student, you can avoid stress and learn more by requesting the help of an expert.

• *To identify the family member who will be most helpful to the patient and/ or facilitate the family's efforts to coordinate care.* This is often difficult, sometimes impossible. The therapist will look for an individual with the following characteristics:

   – Someone who is fond of and in touch with the patient—who may or may not live with the patient

   – Someone who seems respected by and "has the ear of" many in the family

   – Someone who is most often among those who visit the patient (in the hospital) or who accompanies him or her to clinic

   – Someone who is liked and respected by the patient

• *To deliver news that the patient has died or taken a turn for the worse.* Wherever possible, do this in a personal meeting rather than by phone. If a physician or therapist is not available and this difficult task falls to you, you may want to begin directly with "I have some difficult news," or "I regret to tell you . . ." If the death or change in condition has been expected, you may want to say that early in the interaction as well.

- *When the patient's condition is frightening or has a poor prognosis.* Fears and sorrow may surface during a conversation or interview with the family and patient. The therapist can help you identify helpful and nonhelpful patterns of family interaction.

> Working with the family is an integral part of quality patient care. It can have important rewards for the patient, the family, and yourself. They will not always be apparent at the time.

12 Evaluations

Bane or Blessing?

In 1982, 70% of faculty responding to a national survey felt that *contemporary clerkship evaluation did not ensure identification of deficiencies in students' knowledge, skills, and attitudes* (Association of American Medical Colleges, 1982). There is no newer evidence to suggest that these opinions have changed. It is also revealing that three current manuals for students about the clinical years say virtually nothing about clerkship evaluation (Gusky, 1982; Lederman, 1990; Polk, 1995).

In medical education, evaluation provokes considerable anxiety. A vast information pool and extreme emphasis on cognitive material both contribute to this. The grading process is designed to discriminate between students rather than ensuring satisfactory levels of competence for all who graduate. Therefore, many exam questions are obscure, sometimes absurdly so.

In clerkships, three additional factors cloud evaluation: (a) students receive substantially different amounts of ongoing evaluation and feedback; (b) the teachers evaluate significantly "by the seat of their pants"—most are well intentioned and sincere, but few are really good at this; (c) in some clerkships, as Polk (1995) cogently states, "The paradox of ward medicine is its demand that students show maturity they cannot have gained, but for lack of which they still lose points" (p. 28).

How You Will be Evaluated

Some General Comments

On all clerkships, there is sporadic evaluation, supervision, and feedback throughout the clerkship. This will be done by your residents, attending physician, and clerkship director. Nurses and other health care professionals may participate. The amount and quality of such activity and the resultant judgments vary substantially for the following reasons:

- Most are based on unstructured (no format, no criteria) observation of your presentations and write-ups, and the informal quizzes and observations during rounds (see Table 12.1).
- Instructors differ in their degree of sophistication in regard to evaluation; those well trained in such evaluation are still rare.
- Instructors vary in their willingness to hear student presentations on rounds and read student write-ups.

Not surprisingly then, *you and your colleagues in the same clerkship may not be supervised and evaluated in comparable ways.* One student may have two completely supervised physical exams and make a number of new patient presentations. Another may present only once and be casually observed on two or three occasions as he or she listens to a certain heart murmur or examines a skin lesion. The help given you to learn procedures (such as arterial sticks, chest taps, or lumbar punctures) is also extremely variable. The ancient adage, "see one, do one, teach one" still seems to apply.

Such unstructured evaluation can furnish helpful data, but its capriciousness has led to increasing use of recorded anecdotes, behavioral checklists, and standardized observations to make performance evaluation more systematic and structured.

Clinical evaluations may feel subjective (and at times unfair) to you compared with the basic science short-answer exams. This perception is an illusion of medical education. *All evaluation is subjective;* only the format or scoring may be more "objective" in one form of evaluation than another.

About Quizzing

Quizzing on rounds may provide a large part of the hazy, unrecorded database for a student's final evaluation. This is unfortunate because such quizzing

Table 12.1 Clerkship Evaluation

Types of Evaluation	Final Product or Instrument	
Unstructured	*Rating scale*	*Narrative comments*
Write-ups[a]	X	
Presentations	X	X
Quizzing	X	X
Observation during rounds and work periods	X	X
Critical incidents		X
Structured		
Written Exams	Exam scores	
Observation of workup or standardized patient	Rating profile	
Evaluation of write-ups	Written comments based on long-standing implicit or stated explicit criteria	

a. Write-ups may be subject to both structured and unstructured evaluation.

is predominately fact oriented and often trivial rather than an assessment of the critical thinking, problem-solving, or attitudinal processes that are more predictive of your ultimate performance as a doctor.

Critical Incidents

Some clerkship directors and faculty write brief anecdotal reports that reflect student performance. These can be anxiety provoking, but are important and often extremely useful.

Today, while I examined a patient, the medical student, Smith, was interviewing the patient in the next bed. I was impressed with her facilitation of the patient's narrative, her thoughtfulness in suggesting a glass of water, and when the patient was telling how his diagnosis of cancer was established, the student's choice of empathetic words. (An attending physician)

A resident wrote the following anecdote:

At 8:15 am, Cruise, a third-year clerk, drew blood from Mr. Cassidy. He had difficulty finding a vein, refused the patient's suggestion that he get help, and finally after success on the fourth stick, he left the bedside abruptly without apologizing or comforting the patient. Mr. Cassidy was surprised and angry, and several hours later the student had not returned to check the venepuncture sites.

Anecdotes that reflect well on your performance may, via the "dean's letter" (a key item in your residency application) positively influence a residency appointment. If anecdotal reporting is done on your clerkship(s), you can request copies from the clerkship coordinator or your dean of student affairs.

Final Exams

Clerkship evaluation may include a final exam, often a "shelf-copy" written exam from the National Board of Medical Examiners. Simulated clinical problems may be part of it. Your final might also include a structured evaluation during which you are observed and rated while conducting a patient (simulated or real) interview, doing a physical exam, or both. Still far from routine, this is increasingly common. These are called *structured* or *standardized* evaluations because every student is exposed to the same or equivalent problems and rated using the same criteria. Thus, they are more valid than other techniques, particularly casual quizzing.

More About Presentations and Write-Ups

Students appreciate the opportunity to present to attending faculty. Because these verbal summaries reflect the student's ability to relate to and obtain information from the patient, it is essential that faculty accede to this desire.

It's very valuable to learn to present coherently, and the only way you can do that is by doing it [presenting] over and over again and having someone tell you that you missed something. (third-year student)

Often, however, you may not get the opportunity to make full presentations to the attending during rounds.

Due to their length and time pressures on faculty, student write-ups are seldom read in their entirety and some not at all. This is unfortunate. Ask your attending and/or resident to read, at a minimum, the major active problem(s) (present illness), physical examination, problem formulation (your thinking), and master problem list (Chapter 9) in a number of your write-ups chosen sequentially throughout the clerkship. Evaluation of your write-ups may be included as an item in the rating scale. It is more helpful if comments accompany the returned write-up; you learn promptly what needs improvement.

How Evaluative Judgments Are Recorded and What May Go in Your File

Any or all of the ***boldface and italicized*** items discussed below may end up in your file.

Rating scales used on most clerkships (see Appendix 12.1, Sample Rating Scale, at the end of this chapter) usually ask for judgments of your overall performance as well as separate ratings on the skills of history taking, physical exam, rapport with patients, getting "scut" work done, promptness, and (sometimes) appearance.

Faculty members (including house staff) complete these scales at the end and sometimes halfway through the clerkship. They recall the results of informal quizzing and your willingness and proficiency in doing scut work, review "critical incidents," and sift impressions gleaned while observing you at work. They may or may not add narrative comments. If rating scales are carefully constructed and used with other regular feedback, by diligently trained instructors, they can enhance your education. But the judgments requested are often too global ("physical exam skills are excellent, good, fair, poor"), and the criteria (what constitutes "fair," "poor") may not be clearly stated. Some schools use the same rating scale for all clerkships, minimizing the uniqueness of each clerkship. Obviously, no single instrument can fit diverse clerkships and clerkship roles.

Standardized/structured assessments used in the clerkship (if any) may be reflected in the rating scales, but more often they are documented separately. Because the objectives and criteria have been specified, they are usually fair and accurate. If you are supervised in one of these, ask for feedback immediately afterward.

Written exam scores will also figure into your final evaluation.

Anecdotes and critical incidents may not be articulated until a grading session with faculty and perhaps the chief nurse. When used, most incidents will be recalled from memory because few are described in writing. Be sure to ask in advance whether anecdotes or critical incidents are part of your evaluation. Knowing this can diminish inconsistencies and injustices in evaluation but may not weaken the validity of student laments.

Sometimes it only takes one incident, either good or bad to determine your evaluation. If you screw up just once, no one ever forgets. If you shine early, you can't do anything wrong. (third-year student)

Self-Evaluation

Your self-perceptions are very important because they help you set priorities and seek appropriate assistance. **Cultivate the skills of self-evaluation.** They are essential because *in practice you are your own most available judge.* Usually, with repetition and feedback, self-evaluations are accurate. However, many students shy away from systematically profiling their own performance, rationalizing that if "I wasn't doing all right, they'd let me know." This is not a safe assumption.

Activity: Table 12.2 shows a list of things to evaluate yourself on. After filling it out once or twice, particularly if you feel you aren't doing well, ask a resident or an attending to fill it out also and see how your judgments compare with theirs.

Suggestions, Cautions, and Advice

• **Early in the clerkship, get briefed on the evaluation process.** Find out exactly what the evaluation consists of and how the judgments are made. Look at the rating scales and narrative comment forms that will be used, and question anything you don't understand. Clarify the meaning of each item and understand the criteria (if stated) for the various ratings. Learn who performs which evaluations and the role of your clerkship director. He or she can help you negotiate any disparities between your own view of your work and the faculty's.

• **Always ask for feedback after your first two weeks on major clerkships.** Again, review the evaluation forms with the attending, the resident, or both. Your entire student group can do this at once. You may learn that your write-ups are most important to the attendings and the scut work most important to the residents (if you do the scut, the resident is happy, and "a happy resident gives a good evaluation"). Sometimes both perceptions may operate.

Table 12.2   Self-Evaluation Form

Evaluation Item	Rating 1, 2, 3, 4[a]
Industry (willingness to do the work)	
Dependability, trustworthiness	
Level of enthusiasm	
Extent of commitment to clerkship requirements and patients	
How well are you coping with the difficult emotional and spiritual aspects of the experience?	
Your overall level of satisfaction	
Is your fund of knowledge and skills increasing?	
Considering the length of time on this clerkship, rate your level of satisfaction.	
Interviewing	
History taking	
Establishing rapport with patients	
Working effectively with residents and staff	
Physical exam	
Problem formulation	
Assessment and plan	
List any insecurities, pet peeves, stresses.	

a. Rating summaries: 1 = entirely satisfied; 2 = doing well but can improve; 3 = just barely satisfied; 4 = need a lot of help with this.

• **Review evaluations with evaluators.** If the faculty agree, initiate such a review by rating yourself on the forms. See how your ratings compare with faculty ones. You can learn a lot by doing this. Next, review your ratings by faculty and do not hesitate to question ones that seem inappropriate.

> Jim, a clerk on Internal Medicine, asked to see his four-week evaluation forms. He was rated 3 (out of 5) on physical exam skills. He requested clarification. "Well," said the attending, "I watched you listen to a patient's heart for the murmur of mitral stenosis. You didn't turn the patient on his left side." Jim said he did not know that such positioning was important; neither the attending nor resident had mentioned it. "Anything else?" Jim asked. Dr. Important then admitted he could not recall other times when he had actually observed Jim examining a patient. He agreed to change the physical exam rating to read, "insufficient observations."

• *Take criticism seriously.* It is a mistake to be frivolous or discount criticism by deciding the source was incompetent. It is best to assume that unfavorable criticism is valid and explore its meaning with the critic; there is always room for change or improvement. By taking criticism seriously, you will do better in the final evaluation. In the following incident, the student discounted criticism:

> An intern watched a student do a procedure on a patient. The PGY-1 became alarmed with the student's technique and took over. Later, he "read the book" to the student for 10 minutes. Subsequently, the student told a colleague, "Well, Dan (the PGY-1) blew off like a madman for something he does himself and later Ropwan (the PGY-2) spent God knows how long telling me the right way to do it. *Well, I'm more up on the procedure than either of them, and when I get into practice I'll do it my way[!]*" [italics added]

Evaluation is a powerful teaching tool and a critical part of the educational process. Becoming skillful at self-evaluation is essential. Evaluation is also a key factor in your residency applications. It pays to be proactive in ensuring that it is as meaningful and fair as possible. Good luck!

Appendix 12.1. Sample Rating Scale

Northeastern Ohio Universities College of Medicine
FAMILY MEDICINE CLERKSHIP
Student Performance Evaluation: Patient Care
January 4, 2000 - February 11, 2000

Evaluator_____ Date_____

RATING CRITERIA

1	2	3	4	5	X
Unacceptable	Below Expected Performance	Expected Performance	Above Expectations	Consistently Outstanding	Unable to Evaluate

Circle the rating which best describes the student's performance in each skill area below based on what you would expect from a junior medical student. Circle "X" if you are unable to evaluate an area because of insufficient contact with the student.

Please Support All Ratings of "I" and "5" With Specific Comments.

HISTORY TAKING

1	2	3	4	5	X
Superficial, disorganized, incomplete, not focused on patients' problems		Logical, thorough, purposeful, efficient		Consistently well-organized history, guided by thoughtful clinical reasoning and patient needs	

Comments:

PHYSICAL EXAMINATION

1	2	3	4	5	X
Cursory, non-directed, insensitive, awkward, incomplete		Thorough, systematic, accurate		Efficient, considerate of patient's privacy and comfort, directs exam to patient's symptoms	

Comments:

MEDICAL KNOWLEDGE

1	2	3	4	5	X
Insufficient knowledge base, has difficulty integrating textbook knowledge with problem solving and topic presentation		Adequate fund of basic/clinical knowledge, integrates textbook knowledge and clinical experiences		Active in increasing knowledge base that is already above the level of a junior medical student, seeks resources, shares knowledge	

Comments:

ORGANIZING AND RECORDING DATA

1	2	3	4	5	X
Inaccurate, disorganized, irrelevant, illegible, wordy, incomplete		Organized, logical, readable, complete		Consistently discriminates between relevant/irrelevant data, records accurate, concise problem-oriented information	

Comments:

CLINICAL JUDGMENT/DIAGNOSTIC SKILLS

1	2	3	4	5	X
Over reliance on tests, misses major problems, shows premature closure, presents incomplete plans		Identifies/prioritizes problems, generates logical differential diagnoses, is considerate of patient needs, costs		Appropriately copes with uncertainties of ambulatory care, adjusts care to patient's needs	

Comments:

PRESENTATION SKILLS

1	2	3	4	5	X
Is unprepared, presents ineffective, in- complete or irrelevant information		Presents clear, organized, relevant, thoughtful information		Presents appropriate differential diag- noses and treatment plans, is time efficient and adapts presentation style to needs of listeners	

Comments:

ORIENTATION TO FAMILY/COMMUNITY

1	2	3	4	5	X
Routinely ignores obvious family and community issues		Inquires about family/community sup- port and includes this information in case presentations/discussions		Develops management plans with con- sideration of psychosocial factors and the impact of family/community on health care	

Comments:

INTERPERSONAL SKILLS

1	2	3	4	5	X
Is disrespectful, intolerant, lacks empathy/compassion, communicates poorly		Establishes rapport, speaks clearly, uses patient-appropriate vocabulary, shows respect and compassion		Engenders confidence, takes active interest in problems of all patients, keeps patient and family informed and involved	

Comments:

FAMILY MEDICINE PERSPECTIVE

1	2	3	4	5	X
Recites fact, presents all patient prob- lems as initial, urgent, isolated		Occasionally discusses patient problems in context of comprehensive, continuous care		Consistently applies patient problems to comprehensive care, reviews patient's chart in order to provide continuous care	

Comments:

PATIENT EDUCATION/HEALTH PROMOTION

1	2	3	4	5	X
Fails to address health promotion and health risks, avoids patient education opportunities		Discusses health risks associated with the patient's presenting problem, will- ing to provide information to the patient		Remembers to check with the patient or chart about health risks regardless of the reason for the visit, resourceful in providing information to the patient	

Comments:

MOTIVATION/ATTITUDE

1	2	3	4	5	X
Immature, irresponsible, unreliable, unmotivated, unaware of limitations/ problems		Self-motivated, accepts/acts on feed- back, works within limits of knowledge and training		Consistently punctual, available, relia- ble to "go the extra mile" for patients/ colleagues, recognizes and responds to patient needs	

Comments:

**I have reservations about this student's ability to become a competent physician based on his/her clinical skills, interpersonal skills, or professional behav-
ior.   No   Yes, because** _____

SOURCE: This rating scale is shown with the permission of the Department of Family Medicine, Northeastern Ohio Universities College of Medicine. The reverse side of the form (not shown) has sections for rating presentation skills, orientation to family/community, interpersonal skills, family medicine perspective, patient education/health promotion, and motivation/attitudes.

Part III

Major Issues in the Implicit Curriculum

13 Exhaustion, Loneliness, Depression, and Anxiety

Exhaustion, loneliness, depression, and anxiety are frequent comrades in medical training and practice. Although capable of masterful soliloquies, they prefer dialogue or group scenes. They disguise themselves expertly with masks and denial. Their scripts are wooden and uninspired, often aiming at entanglement. You gain an advantage when you accept sleep deprivation and overwork as foster parents to this sullen crowd.

Sleep Deprivation and Exhaustion

Some General Data

Exhaustion is common among medical students on major clinical assignments who spend 50 to 100 hours a week on the service and additional time studying. A person may work from 7 a.m. one day through that night on-call and 10 to 12 hours the next day—more than 34 hours without sleep. Then he or she is due back at work early the next morning. House staff may be stretched even more.

A few years ago in New York City, media stories on medical mistakes aroused concern about the exploitation of house staff. Legislation was passed to limit the hours physicians could work consecutively in the hospital setting.

125

In some Scandinavian countries, the law limits the hours per week a physician can work. The impact of such laws is uncertain.

More widespread is a decrease in the frequency a resident or student must take night call. In clerkships and residencies, "call" every other night used to be commonplace; now it is customarily every third, fourth, or fifth night. Some departments assign a special team to take night call on all of its units.

On any service, it is not unusual to see students or house officers sleep during conferences, nod off during sit-down rounds, or rarely, even at the bedside. Surgical clerks and PGY-1s occasionally fall asleep holding retractors at the operating table.

Sleep and Sleep Deprivation

Sleep is one of our best friends, yet too many working hours rob us of its benefits. Of American adults, 37% are chronically sleep deprived. Drivers falling asleep at the wheel cause many serious accidents. We have known medical students who were killed while driving; circumstances suggested they fell asleep.

Sleep has circadian rhythms controlled by the pineal gland. Superimposed on these rhythms are controls responding to the relative amounts of sleep and awake time in the previous few days. Insufficient sleep raises cortisol (the "stress hormone") levels. Short-term lack of sleep can actually marshal the immune response for a few days, but then it deteriorates. Chronic sleep deprivation will increase your susceptibility to infection. Jet lag may confuse the circadian rhythms of sleep so that we don't rest well when traveling.

Medicine is an error-prone activity; mistakes occur (Hilfiker 1991; Paget, 1998; see also Chapter 5). Inevitably, students who are sleep deprived (and too many are) are more prone to make mistakes. Many of us have poor personal warning systems. We do not always perceive when we are pushing too hard or that our lives are too crowded. We become prey to faulty judgment. Sleep fuels our security system against mistakes. Life is *more* difficult with insufficient sleep.

Activity: Answer the following questions:

1. How many hours of sleep per 24 hours did you average during the last two weeks you were on a major clinical service?
2. Do you ever feel that you are pushing too hard?
3. Do you feel worn out at the end of the day?

4. Which of your pleasures have you forgone in med school (tennis, running, gardening, bridge, reading the paper, etc.).
5. How is the ethic of working hard and sleeping less communicated to you?

Reflect on your answers and discuss them with colleagues.

The seductive aspect of medical work, often combined with a valid (or exaggerated) sense of responsibility, contributes heavily to sleep deprivation. "If I stick around longer, maybe I'll see a case I wouldn't see otherwise," or "We'll start new therapy on Mr. Joslin that I need to know about," or "I'll have a chance to do a procedure I haven't done before." Doing new procedures is compelling. The allure of the seriously ill and the desire to help them is powerful. If you were a "hero" in your childhood, or your altruism is still vibrant, it is particularly hard not to do *more* or to do whatever *for longer,* whether it is absolutely necessary or not. Unquestionably, there are rewards in devoting extra time to challenging patients. The trick is to consider your welfare as well as the patients'.

Loneliness

Loneliness is a subtle, sometimes powerful dimension of clerkships. Often, medical students and house staff assume that because they're working with other people every day, they can't be lonely. Wrong!

Loneliness is engendered by lack of sufficient *meaningful* contact with other people or with one's own inner resources. Because important relationships are at jeopardy in medical school, some of yours may have already been abandoned or weakened. This increases your risk of loneliness. One student bemoaned the difficulty of getting friends to understand "the complete lack of control one has over one's life in third year. Maybe I should tell [my friends] . . . what I had to go through to get out of three hours of surgery when I had been subpoenaed by a Federal court. 'Tell them you're a doctor and you can't go,' my resident told me!" (Coombs, 1998, p. 107).

We have observed people doing their jobs extremely well without meaningful contact with other staff. Doctors interact with one another and, as needed, with nurses and students, and the medical students talk with one another, but virtually every exchange is focused on getting work done. There was no *person-to-person* contact. Although we did not follow everyone home at night, many of these people lived alone or with people whose work was equally demanding. We assume that, in many cases, meaningful interactions were minimal at home also. Regardless, loneliness at work was powerful and often unrecognized by the lonely person.

Anxiety and Depression

In medical students, sleep deprivation definitely contributes to anxiety and depression. There are other roots (see Figure 13.1): academic pressure (including unbridled competitiveness), poor performance, and emotionally difficult events (dying patients, emergencies, any particularly sad, exhausting, or anger-provoking scenario) can all contribute. Personal factors may be involved as well—for example, being away from home, difficulties in a relationship, or lack of exercise. In other instances, depression may be related to the busyness of life and work, to one's need to not be in conflict with others, or to no longer having time for hobbies, art, or other means of self-expression. These are all circumstances for which medical students are at high risk.

> During her surgery clerkship, Gail, a new third-year student, felt particularly anxious—"like things were not OK." When something "went wrong" with an assigned patient, she felt responsible. Gail shared a rental with two other women. Their relationships were pleasant but not accompanied by any real intimacy. It was easy to hide feelings, and she did not share them with other friends either. She felt it was not acceptable for a student doctor to be anxious (or depressed or lonely); therefore, it was a risk to talk about it. She was convinced that the faculty would consider it a weakness and give her a bad grade. Years later, in therapy, she became aware of the true depth of her loneliness during third year.

Most emotionally aware people acknowledge significant depression at various times in their lives. Of course, depression can occur as a natural mood swing during certain situations and transitions. A clerkship might stimulate such a situational depression. Usually, such swings are only a few days or less in duration and not accompanied by signs of organic depression—insomnia, loss of appetite, crying spells, hopelessness, and perhaps thoughts of suicide.

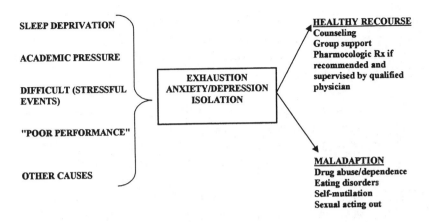

Figure 13.1. Contributors to Depression and Anxiety in Medical Students

Depression in Oneself or a Colleague

When we encounter serious depression, we often try to defuse it in some way and hope it will disappear. Unsubstantiated reassurance (the "pep talk"), distractions (a vacation or an extravagant date), and ignoring are common. It is wiser and healthier to remember that depression may signify a change, loss, or transition that is important to acknowledge, endure, and emerge from—hopefully, richer in some way. It is maddening to hear that something that feels terrible and that can also adversely affect others may be a gift. But eventually, perhaps years later, a period of depression may indeed be appreciated as a font of insight or the stimulus to make a signal life change.

If organic signs of depression are present, particularly if they include suicidal thoughts or plans, it is mandatory to see a psychotherapist who can decide if the depression might respond to counseling or, in this age of "biological psychiatry," antidepressant medication.

Isolation

Isolation is a defense mechanism. Being "perfect," clowning, acting out, joking, and "medication" are others. We use them to insulate ourselves from fear, abandonment, anger, frustration, or other emotional pain.

Isolation and solitude are not the same. Periods of solitude are important for most of us. Most solitude takes place apart from others, but it is a supportive, enriching, often creative experience. Solitude is self-regenerative. Isolation is extreme withdrawal—an unhealthy, self-protective, hiding phenomenon, a stultifying escape from emotional or spiritual pain. In *Gift From the Sea,* Anne Morrow Lindbergh (1955) writes:

> It is not the desert island nor the stony wilderness that cuts you off from the people you love. It is the wilderness in the mind, the desert wastes in the heart through which one wanders lost and a stranger. When one is a stranger to oneself then one is estranged from others too. (p. 44)

The unawareness that can accompany isolation may encourage it as a habitual reaction to poor performance, prolonged uncertainty, depression, and emotional distress. When depressed, we isolate to feel safer, which, in reality, insulates us from help by amputating our channels to nurture and support. Isolation cuts us off from friends and prevents us from developing new ones. One student said, "I feel like I'm at the other end of the world from everybody" (Coombs, 1998, p. 83).

Isolation changes us. It retracts the antennae that tune us in to the feelings of others. It smothers affection. We don't struggle as effectively with isolation as we do with some other aspects of the troubled self. When we are isolating, it is not that we don't reach out; it is more that, until we begin to heal, we can't. In this way, depression and isolation possess us—like fabled evil spirits. The "relief" that isolation provides from emotional pain is as addicting, and in the long term as useless, as many drugs. It seizes us and is often well ensconced before we realize it.

> In his third year, Steve struggled with powerful doubts about "being a doctor" while also contemplating increased commitment to a romantic partner. In therapy, he initially spoke clearly about his feelings; then he didn't show up for several weeks. When he did reappear, he told how his isolation "feeds upon itself," how he was determined "not to contact anyone until I am through this." He acknowledged feeling helpless and of "knowing that I need help but feeling too exposed and raw to even ask for it."

Although he was aware that he was isolating, and how serious it was, he could not break out of it. He had felt unable to emerge; he was ashamed that he had not been in touch. When reminded that support and acceptance are as much the function of the counselor as advice and guidance, he agreed to meet again.

"Medication":
Dealing With the Pain

Although isolation is perceived by the ego as protective, it will not truly assuage emotional pain and discomfort. Further withdrawal or "medication" is sought. Habitual substance use/abuse can accompany or emerge from emotional or spiritual withdrawal and their antecedents—anxiety, depression, and loneliness. If habitual use provides satisfactory numbing, full-scale dependence can result (see Chapter 16). Another common form of "medication" is risky, promiscuous, or disloyal sexual behavior. Sexual/emotional affairs occur among house staff, and medical students. Although some bloom into firm and lasting commitment, more often, they are short-lived. If the sexual activity is habitually related to psychological distress, particularly emotional pain, then sex is probably being used in similar fashion to a drug.

The healthy alternative to "medication" is the fostering of mindful self-care—conscious intervals of attention to one's self and one's sanity: periods of play, relaxation, meditation, exercise, even if brief. See Chapters 15 through 19.

Conclusion

This chapter has dealt with the exhaustion, loneliness, depression, and anxiety that can beset you during intense and difficult clinical work. In *Gaudeamus Igitur (Therefore, let us rejoice)* John Stone, M.D., muses on medical studenthood. The following excerpt is apropos.

> For you must fear ignorance more than cyanosis
> For whole days will move in the direction of rain
> For you will cry and there will be no one to talk to
> or no one but yourself
> For you will be lonely
> For you will be alone
> For there is a difference
> For there is no seriousness like joy
> For there is no joy like seriousness
> For the days will run together like gallops and the years
> go by as fast as the speed of thought
> which is faster than the speed of light

or Superman
or Superwoman
For you will not be Superman
For you will not be Superwoman
For you will not be Solomon
but you will be asked the question nevertheless .."
                                    —*John Stone, M.D. (1991, p. 348)*

14 Death Is the Enemy

O Lord of Mysteries, how baffling, how clueless
is laggard death, disregarding
all that is set before it
in the dignity of welcome—
laggard death, that steals
insignificant patches of flesh—
laggard death, that shuffles
past the open gate,
past the open hand,
past the open,
ancient,
courteously waiting life.

—Denise Levertov (1991, p. 258)

Has anyone close to you died? Have you yet visited the ICU of a busy hospital? Do you know firsthand the family vigil of critical care? Have you agonized over prolonging the life of a loved one who is fatally ill?

The unspoken perspective that "death is the enemy" has great power in the education and practice of physicians, nurses, and other caregivers. Far too much is done to avert death in hopelessly ill patients and far too little time is spent exploring alternatives with family and patients.

We both deplore and understand this. Many writers suggest that awareness of death is mankind's central adult concern, that death anxiety haunts us like

133

nothing else. In *The Denial of Death,* Becker (1973) argues that all of psycho-therapy must be reworked and refigured to acknowledge this central preoccu-pation and cause of suffering.

So not surprisingly, "death is the enemy" reflects these concerns.

Death Is the Enemy:
Impact on Patient Care

The verse opening this chapter is the last stanza of "Death Psalm: O Lord of Mysteries," by Denise Levertov. Earlier verses eloquently describe how an elderly loved one has prepared for death during life. In part: "She remembered her griefs / She remembered her happiness / . . . / She told her sons and daugh-ters she was ready / She maintained her readiness." Then "She grew very old / . . . / She did not die" . . . "and now lies half speechless, incontinent, / aching in body, wandering in mind / in a hospital room." Levertov describes tubes in every orifice, black bed sores, and then says, "She is not whole." The poem concludes with the verse that opens this chapter.

In teaching hospitals, the preservation of life by extreme and costly mea-sures is commonplace. More than 75% of any one person's lifetime health and medical costs is spent in the last 6 to 12 months of life. The perspective that *death is the enemy* fuels this asymmetry. In critical care, the ambience is ur-gency, emergency, and haste. *It is harder to decide to watch someone die than to stay busy keeping them alive.* When, as a participant, you feel confused, it may be hard to find a resident, fellow, or attending to explore the questions with you. They are responding to the demands, *modus operandi,* and culture of the environment. You may adopt the same passive acceptance before completing the rotation. Repeated exposure to these attitudes and response patterns during training can strongly influence the way you eventually practice and teach.

Activity: Considering a recent experience with death/dying how do you respond to Questions 1-3? (Box 14.1) If you have no experience, key your answers to the following case:

Ms. O'Neill, a 92-year-old woman, came to the hospital with jaun-dice and severe abdominal pain. Physical exam and MRI revealed a

---

BOX 14.1

Central Issues Around Death and Dying

1. Is death being unnecessarily and/or inappropriately prolonged?
2. Is what's being done for a given patient reasonable and humane?
3. Were extreme measures adequately discussed? Did we consider added suffering, the likelihood of success, quality of the aftermath, and the emotional, spiritual, and financial cost?
4. How have particular death or dying episodes affected you as a person and as a professional?

---

pancreatic tumor (almost certainly cancer) obstructing the common bile duct. The patient was alert, oriented, febrile (temperature 103° F) and hypotensive. Lab tests also established renal failure and an infection of the bile duct and liver, which had spread to the blood stream. The patient agreed to fluid replacement and antibiotics, but said, "If this is cancer, I want no heroic treatment." She preferred hospice care with adequate pain control, saying that she had lived a long and wonderful life and was entirely ready to die. Her primary internist, however, instituted peritoneal dialysis as well as drugs to raise her blood pressure. The medical student said, "I'm confused. Ms. O'Neill is ready to die, but her physician is fighting her every step of the way."

An infectious disease specialist was consulted. She spent extra time with Ms. O'Neill and established that the patient definitely wanted to stop dialysis and be transferred to hospice care. The primary physician refused that course of action stating, "The patient has good insurance and we will be fully remunerated if she stays in the hospital." In profound disagreement, the infectious disease consultant resigned from the case.

This example is not rare. On oncology services, the administration of heroic (often unpleasant) measures is commonplace. The typical bill for CCU or ICU services is $2,000 to $4,000 a day.

Do We Strive for Healing or "Live Lines?"

Everyone dies—sooner or later. For many in the medical profession, "sooner" is troublesome. As physicians and physicians-in-training, as critical care nurses, it is important to remember that *the highest purpose of our work is not to keep people alive against great odds but to deal with illness effectively and compassionately, to alleviate pain and suffering, to instill reasonable hope, and to halt or cure disease when we can.*

Obviously, for many patients, it makes sense to prolong life with reasonable or even heroic measures. For someone still capable physically and/or intellectually and/or spiritually, who wants to live and who has the potential for loving and supporting others or doing productive work, we must do our best. Saving life will reasonably ensure further quality time. But sometimes in the CCU or ICU, one feels that doctors and nurses treat monitors, not patients, that "live lines" on the screen matter most, and that the staff feels defeated when the lines go flat. We must devote our energy to well-considered ethical and moral choices, not "battles" against the flat line.

Suggestions. Periodically, discuss Questions 1 through 3 in Box 14.1 with the patient (when possible), colleagues, and the patient's family. Keep asking yourself, your teachers, your colleagues, and the family, "Does it feel like we're doing the best thing."

For patients who choose to abandon further extreme measures, Box 14.2 offers some ways you can help them.

Death:
Impact on the Caregiver

Physicians experience deaths among their patients. On some services, particularly critical care, deaths may be frequent. Despite detachment (Chapters 16, 18), these deaths affect you. If you had a meaningful relationship with the patient, his or her death will constitute a significant loss. If you are also psychologically enmeshed by "death is the enemy," your esteem and competence are sullied in your own eyes. Not only is your spirit affected if the patient dies, but your professional competence comes under question, more so if different treatment choices might have changed the course of events. *Most often, the questioner is yourself.*

BOX 14.2

Bringing Comfort and Solace to the Dying Patient

- Listen and reflect: Reflection includes paraphrasing to check out your comprehension and interpretation of what's being said.
- Plan in terms of what the sick person and the family want and need (the "goals"), not what the disease requires.
- Ask, "How can I support you?"
- Reassure the patient about real things, even if small.
- Facilitate work with family, friends, partners.
- Help the patient or his or her surrogate(s) choose the place of death.
- Touch the patient appropriately; hold his or her hand.
- Give your full attention and say little.
- Ask if the patient would like to tell you what this is like for him or her.
- Be clear that the patient will control the pain medication.
- Promote comfort in other ways: "Do you want to see a minister or priest?"
- Help the patient set realistic goals.
- Help clarify and discuss the patient's fears.
- Minimize suffering

Caring for a terminal patient is strenuous and draining. We are not immune to the sorrow involved, and depending on our emotional investment, we can also suffer varying amounts of grief, including anger and helplessness. Yet on busy critical care units, our sorrow is unacknowledged, and we do little or nothing, explicitly, to grieve. To complicate matters, part of you, particularly in the case of the comatose, noncommunicative patient requiring a lot of attention, may want the patient to die. This is seldom discussed.

The effects of such episodes are cumulative. Your first experiences with dying patients are textured by any previous *personal* experiences with death. With time, each new experience is increasingly influenced by prior *professional* experiences rather than personal ones. Thus, diminished emotional responsiveness—the diffidence of doctoring—may dampen or snuff out your reactions (Chapter 16).

So the following scenario might occur. On your first day of service, you inherit two patients in unrelenting pain, both terminal with end-stage cancer. The next morning, a patient your own age is admitted with a far advanced fatal illness. You are also scheduled to talk with the desperate family of a fatally ill loved one. Although you may feel inured to the emotional impact of these events and answer (as the characters are constantly doing on medical TV shows), "I'm OK" to the query, "How are you?" *it may be that you're not really OK.* Your reservoir of secret, emotionally laden, unprocessed matters is bulging. It can burst unexpectedly, often silently, flooding you with sorrow and depression, sleeplessness, nightmares, abusive language, or gallows humor. If it is not defused, such pressure increases your risk for "medicating" in unhealthy ways (Chapters 13, 16).

> Richard W., a 26-year-old fourth-year student, was on the medical service at County Hospital on Christmas Eve. A young man, 28, entered with a rare cancer that had been treated for months with minimal success. He was married with two small children. He was in severe pain and had spent three weeks in another hospital on chemotherapy and analgesics. "They withheld pain medication when I needed it," he reported. He had exhausted his financial resources and was transferred to County Hospital. Richard identified strongly with the patient, felt helpless to comfort him, and was angry that this was happening on Christmas Eve. Although he was off the next day, Richard knew, "I wouldn't be able to forget his bleeding and tortured body. Then," he continued, "the patient's wife and two children arrived. It was more than I could bear."

> The patient, Richard, and the patient's wife all knew he was there to die a miserable, highly premature death. He had no hope. Richard himself had nowhere to turn with his fear, anger, and inadequacy. It was a lose-lose situation on Christmas Eve—a scene of incredible frustration and sorrow. That night, and for weeks afterward, Richard "hated medicine, regretted my decision to become a doctor, and wanted only to go home and drink."

Richard told this story *for the first time eight years later.* The memories were still vivid.

You will find yourself in similar situations. Such scenarios wreak emotional and spiritual devastation on patients and their families. The effects that such experiences have on you are also traumatic. No matter what your age, sex, and prior experience, these circumstances can tax even well-supported and emotionally mature students. It is essential to know where and how to "process" such an event and how to help the patient—especially how to reduce his or her suffering. See Box 14.2 and Chapter 16 for some suggestions you might follow.

We are seldom taught other ways of bringing solace besides curing the disease or that hope about little things is better than no hope at all. It never occurred to Richard that his patient might have found comfort in being invited to talk about his feelings. Or calmed by the knowledge that pain relief was a top priority.

The next story embodies a number of contrasts, some to Richard's tale and some to that of Mrs. O'Neill, told earlier.

Dr. M., a retired physician, was 66 when he began to notice difficulty in saying certain words. Close friends said he "sounded like he had one too many." Over a few months, his speech became more garbled, and he had difficulty swallowing. CT scans and MRIs were negative. Over several more months, he became mute and required a gastrostomy tube through which he hydrated and fed himself. An active gardener and consummate handy man, he continued all his activities and communicated in writing. His spirits remained high and his outlook realistic. To a friend he said, "I am not afraid to die; every month is a gift." By this time the diagnosis of bulbar amyotrophic lateral sclerosis ("Lou Gehrig's disease") was made. Difficulty raising secretions and spells of a racking cough necessitated a tracheotomy, which he has managed well. Dr. M. has a loving and spirited wife of 45 years, four children, and 12 grandchildren. They all live within four blocks. The tracheotomy episode stimulated the family to talk with him about hospitalizations and extreme measures in the future. They agreed that if he gets pneumonia—not unlikely—he will not be hospitalized and a respirator will not be used; he will receive antibiotics and other measures at home. His family and friends have begun to make their farewells. Dr. M.'s spirits remain excellent, and the grace and dignity with which he lives inspires all who spend time with him.

Accepting Death (as a Natural Event)

While by no means the complete answer, **it will benefit physicians and students alike to shift their perspective from** "death is the enemy" (and therefore "my main job is to prevent this person from dying,") **to "some of my patients will die"** (and therefore, "it is part of my work to provide comfort and support in whatever time they have left"). This attitudinal shift will make you more supportive to patients and also provide a more peaceful venue in which to work.

How do you make this shift?

- Reassess your own life priorities and your beliefs and values about death.
- Learn to better identify patients' suffering and how to respond to it (Chapter 16).
- Participate in a support or discussion group. Make it habitual to talk with other professionals about critical care and ethical decisions.
- Learn about your patients' spiritual beliefs and practices in a nonintrusive fashion and help use those beliefs and practices in their healing. Try to intuit what being with this particular person at this particular time in your life is giving you and what you can offer him or her. What is that person's gift to you? Sometimes it is simply the energy you feel from your patient—his or her courage, grace, anger. Often, it is an affirmation, perhaps disguised in a story your patient tells or something he or she brings you to read.

15 Loss of Intellectual Vitality

Education is the acquisition of the art of the utilization of knowledge.
—*Alfred North Whitehead (1957)*

This chapter discusses students' intellectual vitality—a state of robust and flexible intellectual activity. Its salient characteristics are curiosity, creativity, the capability for divergent thinking, integrative capacity, and tolerance for ambiguity. In medicine, it also includes astute medical problem solving and the ability to evaluate clinical research reports. If you endured a premedical program where memorization of facts was the rule, depletion of your intellectual vitality began there. If you attended a college that stimulated and nurtured your intellect, most science courses in medical school were a backward step.

The "Preclinical Lesion"

The odds are high that your biological and behavioral science courses in medical school with their volumes of material, emphasis on small, frequently trivial, pieces of information, a predominantly lecture mode, and the use of frequent multiple-choice exams, all contributed to a "cognitive cookbook" learning experience.

141

Almost any idiot can learn what we have to learn in basic sciences—all
you have to do is memorize; it bothers me that there's not more thinking;
with the right terms, any eighth grader could memorize the same bugs and
drugs we have to memorize. (second-year student)

Comparing it with college, another student declared that medical school
"turned up the gain on trivia." Edward Rodzinski estimates that first-year medical students must memorize upward of 20,000 pieces of factual information
(personal communication, John Engel). He adds, wryly, "What's even more
disturbing is that they do." And Larry Weed, M.D., architect of problem-oriented charting, has repeatedly observed that medical students are asked to
memorize all the answers before they ever know what the questions are.

Certainly, students need to know at least some moderate segment of the basic material. But for neophytes, defining an essential knowledge base without
guidance is an impossible task.

I tried to learn everything and I just couldn't. Now I try to figure out what
they're going to test me on and learn that. . . . it's a bitter pill; it goes
against my values to study for grades. (second-year student)

And so, we believe it is for most students; the "essential" material becomes
what they decide will be on the next test.

In basic science courses, little time is available for creative thinking, identification and discussion of critical questions, or problem solving. It is eat (memorize), regurgitate (test), eat more (memorize), regurgitate again (exam). The
process might be called "academic (or informational) bulimia."[1] "Swallow it
(information), but before you can digest it, vomit it up so we can put more in."

Thus, many students feel deadened by the first two years, "demoralized by a
diminishing sense of intellectual giftedness." In addition, they note the failure
to explore, practice, and encourage thought processes (problem solving, self-
evaluation) and the lack of attention to emotional and spiritual issues.

Fortunately, problem-based learning (PBL) has gained a foothold in the first
and second year of some medical schools. PBL fosters problem-solving skills,
creativity, and curiosity. It is attentive to the methods of patient appraisal and
diagnosis. When used with integrity for teaching problem-solving skills and
emphasizing process and method (and not just as a different format for organizing facts and concepts), it can slow or prevent the decline of intellectual
vitality during Years 1 and 2.

Intellectual Vitality and Clerkship Education

Clerkship education, although not explicitly committed to promoting intellectual vitality, can arrest or reverse the intellectual torpor of first and second year. To your delight, patients will provide context for a significant amount of the basic science material memorized in Years 1 and 2. Now it can be *learned!*

However, the task of staying intellectually alive is still urgent and difficult. The educational process in most clerkships is too thin. Opportunities to promote creativity, increase sensitivity to others, see problems not labels, and to systematically problem solve, are often squandered by faculty. *Most important, the framing, formulation, and illumination of critical questions*—ones that could lead to better care of the patient or that could advance knowledge— *is not often encouraged.* The characteristics of intellectual vitality may not be valued or considered in the grading process. As a result, you can feel defeated, no longer gifted, and that your intellectual traits are underused.

The job is learning enough of this material that I will be able to do medicine without danger to my patients, while learning to relate to them as well. I don't have time to be creative, to pursue special interests or challenges. My interest in people has not been nurtured. I have not learned much about how to do that. (third-year student)

Activity:

1. List three or four creative opportunities you didn't attempt in Years 1 and 2 because of your study load.
2. Recall two recent situations in which you were not OK (emotionally or physically), yet when asked, your reply was "I'm fine."
3. Recall a time as a student (at any level) when you felt positive about both what you were learning and how you were learning it.

Cognitive-Affective Imbalance

So in most clerkships, the dynamic of cognitive-affective imbalance again operates. The processes involved are diagrammed in Figure 15.1. The major focus of rounds, informal conferences, lectures, and examinations is highly specific cognitive material: pathophysiology and description of disease, points

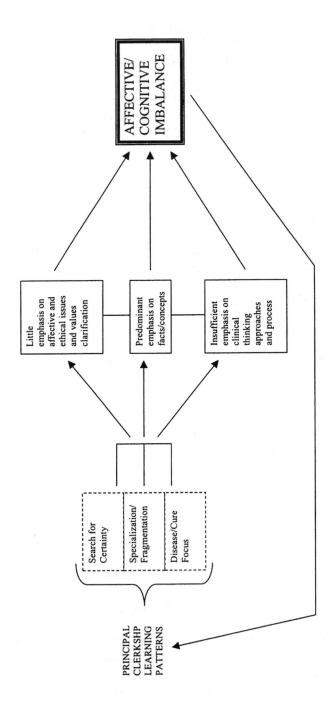

Figure 15.1. Cognitive-Affective Imbalance

of diagnosis, the meaning of tests, treatment, and management. If you are assigned to a subspecialty unit for a major specialty clerkship (e.g., to cardiology for internal/medicine) and/or your attending is a subspecialist, a reductionistic subspecialty perspective may reinforce this cognitive dominance. Many subspecialists are also good generalists, but if their attention is directed to subspecialty problems, they may not reveal the broader underlying orientation you need.

Getting the right answer rapidly is encouraged. Often, it would be more valuable to ask, "What other possibilities did you consider?" or "What questions did this raise for you?" than to move quickly on to the next "short-answer question." The importance of acknowledging and accepting "mystery" and uncertainty are underplayed. *There is strong emphasis on what is "known," whereas uncertainty goes unadmitted or undiscussed.* The game of "pearl dropping" also contributes to the cognitive emphasis (see Chapter 10).

> Sometimes it is overwhelming. . . . You think, I should know this or I should know that. . . . I'm a little bit amazed at even how much the second-year residents know. . . . It's overwhelming, and I wonder, am I ever going to learn all that stuff? (third-year student)

Because the student is an integral part of the workforce, the demanding workload contributes to this odd learning situation. It creates a *do more* mindset, leaving little time for thinking.

The Quick-Fix Mentality and Intellectual Vitality

A consumer-based obsession with the "quick fix" also contributes to diminished intellectual vitality. Television, the Sunday newspaper, and the Internet attest to the huge role of pharmaceutical companies and their advertising colleagues in perpetuating the quick fix. Commercials tell us how medications unfailingly (apparently) provide prompt relief without adverse effects. The pill is king. In Huxley's *Brave New World,* everyone takes "Somex," an antianxiety drug that increases productivity and reduces stress in the workplace. A huge jar of Somex is accidentally overturned at a large conference, spilling hundreds of pills on the floor. Like gulls scrapping for offal, the listeners desert the speaker to scramble on their knees for an adequate supply of pills.

If the pill is king, the procedure is crown prince. Coronary artery by-pass is now among the most common major surgical procedures. Expensive CT scans have become an arm of defensive medicine. Endoscopy of various organs and structures is frequent partly because endoscopy procedures are well reimbursed.

The technology of "fixing" is truly wonderful. The benefits of many medicines and procedures are without question. It is the complicity of physicians and the medical establishment in the thoughtless, defensive, frequently reflex use of drugs and procedures that is alarming. Long before the knowledge explosion, Osler (1995) said, "Remember how much you do not know. Do not pour strange medicine into your patients" (p. 33).

The Role of Managed Care

Has managed care influenced our intellectual vitality? Under managed care, the propensity has escalated to pay for tangible or "hard" patient management strategies and not pay for "talking time" and patient education ("soft" strategies). The payoff is in rapid diagnosis and treatment of disease or injury, not the management and healing of illness and suffering. If the condition is complex and elusive, the payouts are for diagnostic blood tests and endoscopies, which when used appropriately, should be paid for. But for the art of medicine, physicians receive little. The time spent talking and listening—unearthing and sorting the complexities and nuances of chronic abdominal pain, a marriage gone sour, an adolescent who is acting out, or in exploring the lifestyle that preceded the heart attack—is rarely reimbursed. Consequently, many physicians don't embark on these important minutes, thereby losing hours rich in intellectual stimulation.

Managed care also dims the physician's intellectual vitality through the extra time and frustrations required to deal with the system. For example, even when treatment for mental health and drug-related problems is covered in a patient's contract, it is difficult to get authorization. This occurs despite evidence that treatment decreases visits to emergency rooms and reduces health care costs in other ways. Some physicians spend hours each week attempting to get appropriate treatments authorized.

Detecting Intellectual Stagnation

What will warn you of intellectual deadening?

- *First,* your reading, already limited by workload and personal responsibilities will suffer. Suddenly, you aren't reading journal articles about your patients at all.

BOX 15.1

Self-Care:
Specific Suggestions for Averting Intellectual Stagnation

- *Work to define critical questions.* A group of five third-year students organized their own symposium on hypertension. Citing selected literature, each student presented (20 minutes) on preselected topics (pathophysiology, pharmacotherapy, natural history of hypertension, role of sodium and diet, diagnostic tests) and posed important unanswered questions.

- *Spend time exploring specific patient-related issues in medical journals or on the Internet.* Students usually find this stimulating.

- *Don't berate yourself for what you don't know even if it seems critical.* The best doctors are not encyclopedias; they learn what's necessary to meet emergencies in their particular setting, *and* they have a systematic way of approaching, identifying, and resolving clinical problems.

- *Ask a lot of questions.* Learning begins when the right questions are asked. Inquire about points that puzzle you. Ask others what they think the important unanswered questions are. *There are no dumb questions!*

- *Second,* your interest in deriving critical questions is atrophied or paretic.

- *Third,* your curiosity about specific problems is diminished. You have no interest in how lasix works or why sinusitis doesn't consistently produce fever.

- *Fourth,* your creativity is blunted—and not only with respect to medicine.

- *Fifth,* you rely more frequently on the quick fix to certain problems. In outpatient family medicine, for example, you might use antibiotics in upper-respiratory infections more routinely than before.

Despite the discouraging tone of our remarks *it is possible to do clerkships without further compromise of intellectual vitality* and actually regain some ground. There are many intriguing problems before you; critical questions will emerge. In Box 15.1 are specific suggestions to counter loss of intellectual vitality. A self-care box for affective blunting (in Chapter 16) and Chapter 17 will also be helpful in preserving intellectual vitality.

Clerkships may help you escape from the intellectual lethargy of Years 1 and 2, but all too often, there isn't time for much intellectual stimulation. And *that's the paradox. Students and house staff need time to be alive intellectually. The medical care/education process as usually practiced disallows that kind of time.*

Your intellect needs to be challenged. If it is unused, boredom, fatigue, cynicism, and grief can ensue. *You suffer.* If not countered or processed in healthy ways, these phenomena contribute to impairment—including alcohol and other drug abuse, sexual acting out, compulsive eating problems, and too frequently, a callous disregard for patients.

Note

1. Bulimia is an eating disorder in which the patient regularly induces vomiting after a large intake of food—in severe cases after any intake of food.

16 Emotional Unresponsiveness

In a sense, I became anesthetized. I became part of the group, and in some ways, you were proud of your ability to stand it. In other ways, there's something wrong with your ability to stand it. . . . I can't relax. Just like I can't feel anything. If I don't want to feel the bad stuff, then I have to lose the good stuff as well. . . . I don't want to be unfeeling. I don't want to be an unkind, uncaring, unsympathetic person.

—Third-year student

The current public disenchantment with doctors and the medical establishment is attributed, in part, to the emotional rigidity and opacity of many physicians. Moreover, unhealthy emotional adaptation among medical students and residents is an important, little acknowledged root of impairment. Finally, neither miserly reserve nor ebullient emotional expression is compatible with gratifying medical work. Personality traits, family conditioning, and social background notwithstanding, *the intensity of your medical school experiences and the culture of medical training can powerfully influence your emotional responsiveness.*

149

Development of
Diminished Emotional Responsiveness

Preclinical Conditioning

In Chapter 15, we discussed the concept of cognitive-affective imbalance. Facts, pieces of information, and concepts dominate early medical school courses. Emotional experiences, even when salient, are often minimized or neglected entirely. Gross anatomy is a startling example. The names, locations, and relationships of organs and other anatomical structures are taught and emphasized. The emotional experience of confronting (often for the first time) dead bodies and dissecting (i.e., mutilating) them is given little attention. Death and mutilation stimulate fears and sadness. Anxieties about death are common and powerful among anatomy students. Other fears are also abundant (Finkelstein, 1986).

As first- and second-year students, the autopsy suite; laborious, sometimes harsh teaching techniques; and early disturbing, clinical experiences may have also strongly aroused your emotions. Help to process these feelings was negligible or nonexistent. As one student said, "From cadavers to people who are dying, there tend to be a lot of things which are a shock."

Clinical Conditioning

Now, on major clerkships, you will frequently be a protagonist in events of powerful emotional force. You will witness illness, disfigurement, suffering, and death. You will work with patients who are hostile, manipulative, seductive, or even repulsive. You will order and execute procedures that are invasive and painful. As in anatomy lab, no explicit support helps you assimilate and cope with these difficulties. To defend yourself, you will, or are likely to, act as if such experiences are not, in fact, emotionally charged. *You may "de-emotionalize" and unconsciously assume a protective veneer.* In relation to invasive procedures, for example, students had this to say:

I remember the times I was drawn for blood or whatever and I don't like it and it hurts, but when I think of a patient, for some reason, I don't get the impression it's really hurting them.

You become hardened to it [painful procedures on patients] right away. Especially if you know it has to be done. You block it out basically, at least I do.

These students were both reflective and self-aware. Frequently, students are completely unaware of such changes in themselves. Students who are aware of the feelings and changes may choose not to express them, fearful of being considered unfit for medicine. Thus, as a rule, powerful (psychic) stimuli are paired with norms of silence. That is, they are infrequently mentioned or considered by faculty, and systematic processing of them, as in a support group, seldom occurs.

This de-emotionalization has been called "detached concern" (Lief & Fox, 1963) and deemed by some as normative and helpful. We prefer to call it *affective blunting* or *diminished emotional responsiveness,* highlighting our bias that it constitutes a disproportionately weak response to difficult emotional or spiritual stimuli. Blunting interferes with an appropriately full doctor-patient relationship and distorts the student's own emotional life, as the opening quotation for this chapter dramatically illustrates.

Defining Diminished Emotional Responsiveness

Diminished emotional responsiveness or affective blunting includes one or both of the following:

- *Impaired or severely restricted ability to feel one's own anger, sadness, fear, anxiety, and other strong emotions, and/or to deal with them in healthy ways.* Those who "stuff" their emotions are a common example.
- *Decreased or absent capability to "be with the patient"; that is, to acknowledge, be open to, and work effectively with the emotional and spiritual needs and reactions of patients*

Affective blunting is taught or reinforced by three features of the training process:

1. Most house staff behave in this way.

2. When a student explores an emotional, family, or social aspect of a patient's illness, the effort is seldom fully acknowledged. Sometimes, his or her efforts are treated with derision.

3. On rounds and in conferences, "hard" factual issues are discussed; the emotional/spiritual material is too often treated as unimportant. This contributes powerfully to "hardening of the heart" (see below).

The Effects of
Affective Blunting on Patient Care

Depersonalization, Objectification, and Other Effects
on Patient Care

- *A patient's legitimate emotional and spiritual needs are more likely to be discounted or avoided.* Your fear of "difficult emotionality" in patients may also cause you to tune out their concerns. Such discounting leads, at the least, to dissatisfaction, but many patients feel anger and frustration, which can emerge in odd and nonproductive ways.

- *Students (and house staff) often give insufficient attention to the "manners" of patient care.*

One clerkship observer noted, "We sometimes saw students and house staff talk with patients and ignore any visitors present, perform procedures on patients during meals, interrupt telephone conversations without apology, and, occasionally, wake new nonemergency admissions in the middle of the night to complete histories and physicals."

- *Students and house staff can overlook an emotional component that engendered the patient's health problem.* Mis-"cued" by student(s) and residents, an attending may miss it too.

A 35-year-old female came to the office complaining of moderately severe, throbbing headaches with some nausea occurring irregularly over two months. A thorough examination was nonrevealing. Because the headaches were quite troublesome, an MRI (glossary) of her head was ordered. This was normal. The headaches were partially relieved by treatment for migraines. On her third follow-up visit, while chatting with the nurse, she revealed her turmoil and fear over an impending move to another state for her husband's new job. The move had been decided on a week before her headaches began. Following two visits to a therapist where she talked about her fears and resentments, her headaches ceased.

We believe affective blunting is at the root of complaints such as, "I can't relate to my doctor. He's such a cold fish." Or "My doctor treats me like a thing, not a person." And "I just feel awkward in front of my physician." Individual physicians may be unaware of this aspect of their *persona* or minimize how it affects their connection with patients. Even the hale, hearty, and sympathetic bedside manner can, when facile, create distance by preventing doctor and patient from working together effectively on the sadness, undertones, and suffering of the patient's illness.

The Neglect of Suffering

Yet another way to understand the frequent empathic failure of physicians is to consider *suffering*.[1] We are familiar with its most rudimentary definition, to "endure death, pain, or distress." Although prone to think of pain and suffering as synonymous, we can easily summon up examples of pain without suffering and suffering not primarily associated with pain. Chronic osteoarthritis may be painful without either the apprehension or limitations that could cause suffering. In contrast, the young mother with a seriously abnormal Pap smear may have no pain whatsoever but suffer intensely with fear of her uncertain condition. Thus, there is a more compelling meaning to suffering. It is *distress associated with threats to the intactness of the person.* Moreover, suffering is predominately subjective to the patient and wrapped in the meaning he or she gives to his or her illness or injury. This can be known only through careful inquiry. Too often, medical workers ignore or fail to recognize these opportunities.

Identifying Patient Suffering. A patient comes to us suffering in various ways—some related to his or her illness, some to other aspects of existence. The patient may suffer simply from being in a hospital or from the treatment itself. Take time with each patient to determine whether he or she suffers and, if so, the reasons. Remember, minor complaints may be clues that there is profound suffering. If possible, talk with extremely ill or dying patients while they are still able to converse clearly.

Here is a partial list of common causes of suffering, some physically painful but others for which profound distress is uncoupled from the physical:

- The unknown: What is the diagnosis? What happens next? How much pain will I experience? Is there a possibility of dying?

- Pain—especially of an unknown or a known and dreaded cause, such as cancer; untreated or poorly treated pain; once relieved, will it come back?
- Other physical discomforts—bloating, itching, nausea, vomiting, prolonged hunger, sleeplessness, and prolonged fatigue
- Bodily changes—loss of weight, strength, hair, mobility, faculties, senses, and other common capabilities
- Poor communication with physicians or support system
- Care not coordinated; no one person in command or coordinator not available to patient
- Goals of treatment not explicit and/or not discussed with patient
- Long waits between decisions to do something, getting it done, and getting the results
- Disruptions in relationships
- How are family members doing without me? Will I be able to care for them when I go home?

Barriers to Dealing With Suffering. Norms often tell patients, "Don't suffer" or "Suffer through" or "Don't complain about your suffering." This is one of the main barriers to the relief and prevention of suffering. Another is the caregiver's failure to comprehend and/or alleviate a patient's suffering.

For you the students, the deterrents to dealing fully with a patient's suffering include the following:

- Seemingly insufficient time and energy for cogent inquiry
- Feeling inept at such personal inquiry
- Fear that if you succeed in identifying real suffering, you will be unequipped to resolve it
- Evoking emotions the student-physician wants to avoid

But no matter! **Quality patient care requires empathic communication about suffering and sincere and conscientious attempts to alleviate it.** *There is vastly diminished satisfaction in medical work if patients' suffering is private and unmet.*

Effects of Emotional Unresponsiveness on Students and House Staff

Affective blunting can change or rigidify the way you react to your own feelings and the feelings of others.

Your true feelings may become masked by cynicism or indifference, often manifested in disrespectful language and behavior or by gallows humor. Here is an observation by a third-year resident about student (and resident) behavior.

> Another aspect of caring for the patient disturbs me to no end. It's infused in the students within three weeks; that's how they talk about their patients. Here's a student who has been waiting six years to get a patient [and] they're already calling the patient "a hit." They "got another hit from the ER," "got another GI bleeder. . . ." Now I blame the house staff because that's exactly the language [we] use.

Students say that the crunching load, relentless time pressures, and the need to perform well academically leave little time to think or feel about anything else. In extreme situations, students can develop the classical symptomatology of Post Traumatic Stress Disorder (Finkelstein, 1986).

The emotional painfulness of certain patient scenarios plus the predominately cognitive teaching emphasis eventuates in "hardening of the heart." Many clinical teachers employ a teaching dynamic that promotes hardening of the heart. At first, when you interact with patients you are open to both factual data ("head" energy) and the emotional and spiritual material ("heart" energy). You are energized in both realms. Your teacher, however, is interested only in the factual material, so you are left with tension in your "heart place." With your next patient, you again interact with both head and heart. Again, the instructor discusses primarily the cognitive material, and your "heart tension" mounts. In reaction, your "heart wall" thickens, and eventually, after N episodes, your own interactions with patients exclude or minimize heart material. Hardening of the heart defends you against further heart pain. *You no longer solicit emotional and spiritual input from your patients.*

Affective blunting can have major consequences for you professionally and personally by insulating you from your own feelings and those of others. Such diminished emotional responsiveness with hardening of the heart is, perhaps, the main occupational hazard of physicians. It is a paradox: People enter medicine for economic security, intellectual challenge, or most often, because they believe they will be happiest working with and helping people. However, the emotional and spiritual challenges of medicine too often spawn a self-protective shell that not only flaws your patient care but also seriously impedes the development of quality personal (nonprofessional) relationships and family life.

The emotionally parsimonious caregiver may extend that behavior into his or her personal life. Isolation in the face of strong and aversive psychological stimuli may compound an "unresponsiveness." You may turn away from a partner or friend who could help you deal in a healthy way with the emotional side of your work.

These phenomena can demoralize the most supported and emotionally mature physician. As a doctor, you must know how to support your patients and their families—and how you personally can "process" difficult scenarios. **It is imperative that you have the tools and determination to care for yourself** (see Box 16.1 and Part IV).

Patients can stimulate certain defense mechanisms in you that are antithetical to full doctor-patient relationships. The following story illustrates how a conscientious, person-oriented doctor unwittingly blocked certain patient disclosures:

> A year after entering a small group practice, Dr. K underwent a contractual evaluation by his colleagues. To his own and his colleagues' surprise, four patients had complained on the practice's feedback forms about his "cold fish" approach. His partners discounted these comments, but Dr. K called in the dissatisfied patients and asked them directly about their criticisms. Three of the four patients had been on the verge of discussing private emotionally painful situations when Dr. K "interrupted" with three or four rapid-fire medical questions. Puzzled, because he had been sensitized to this flaw in medical school, Dr. K went to a therapist. Together, they unearthed a facet of each patient's story that recalled a similar, painful, long forgotten, episode in Dr. K's own life.

The points above highlight the serious nature of decreased emotional responsiveness. As students, you are expected to find your own way through this

---

BOX 16.1

Self-Care:
Suggestions for Avoiding and
Minimizing Affective Blunting

- **Acknowledge that you're in a risky environment:** It's hard to maintain full emotional responsiveness.

- **Monitor yourself: Talk regularly about specific events.** Stay aware of your feelings. Don't isolate or clam up. Talk with individuals you trust (partner, designated buddy, counselor, mentor) and/ or a support group. You will resist doing this at first. Remember, confide but don't broadcast.

- **Keep an eye on important relationships:** with partner, spouse, kids, family, close friends. Are they more strained? Are you isolating or on a "short fuse" with anyone? If so, you may be closing down, stretched too far, or both. See Chapter 18 for more on preserving relationships.

- **Try to be "with" the patient** and his or her family to the limits of your ability—don't *do to* them and leave. Dr. William Carlos Williams has said there is "peace of mind that comes from adapting the patient's condition as one's own to be struggled with toward a solution" (Williams, 1991, p. 73). You will gain in both compassion and rapport.

---

complex maze. You will often perceive that faculty and house staff see no value in processing emotionally charged material. Many students speak of consciously acquiring diminished emotional responsiveness to help them adapt— to "get used to it." One said "let them change me enough to protect me but not enough to kill me." Another said, "If I don't want to feel the bad stuff, then I have to lose the good stuff as well."

Activity: Every few days, quickly draw a picture of your mood. Reflect feelings in your colors and strokes. Label the drawing with event(s) that provoke the feelings. Save them. "What you draw is less important than how you draw it."[2]

Caregiver Impairment

Although personality characteristics and family, ethnic, and cultural factors also operate, the patterns you develop to cope with the negative aspects of the educational process and the vicissitudes of clinical medicine—especially your own unprocessed emotional/spiritual pain—can contribute to impairment. Table 16.1 shows that physician impairment ranges widely from common, usually less striking manifestations (such as inattention, affective blunting, and carelessness) to less common entities (such as drug abuse or dependence and suicide) that are more overtly disabling and dangerous. Wounds such as the early loss of a revered parent, discounting by parents, abuse, and abject poverty can be powerful contributors. Some assuage the summative psychic pain with various substances or behaviors. Alcoholism, for example, occurs in 8% to 10% of physicians and is often, for a time, carefully masked. Warner is someone whose alcohol dependency was hastened by the strain and traumata of clinical medicine:

> Warner, a 26-year-old PGY-1, enjoyed alcohol a few times during medical school but was never drunk. In internship, he worked 90 to 100 hour weeks, watched young adults die of polio, and constantly treated severe trauma and illness. Within six months, he was drinking heavily at monthly parties and had two glasses of sherry on his nights off before succumbing to sleep. Except for his wife, he had no support system. He quickly became alcohol dependent and, after six years, depressed and suicidal. Only after he began psychotherapy, did he appreciate how the emotional pain of his work contributed to his alcoholism.

Thus, caregiver impairment is a complex problem that speaks to the frequency of poor emotional and spiritual adaptation among physicians—as much an emotional and spiritual phenomenon as a behavioral abberancy.

Health care professionals and students must help identify impaired or possibly impaired colleagues—house staff, attendings, nurses, and medical students. If you believe someone is impaired (see Table 16.1), unethical, mentally disturbed, or misuses alcohol or other drugs (look for poor attendance, inattention, weight loss, unexplained sleepiness, depression, rage, and daytime drinking), express your concerns through channels that guarantee your anonymity. In Warner's case, many colleagues knew he was addicted to alcohol, but not

Table 16.1 An Expanded View of Physician Impairment

Common		*Uncommon*
Affective numbing	Loss & decreased quality of relationships	
	Excessive need for control and/or to please others	"Difficult Doc"
	Misuse, abuse, & addiction to alcohol & other drugs	Other dependencies and addictions
Carelessness and inattention	Hiding errors	Frequent errors
Sleep deprivation and chronic fatigue		
Workaholism		
Low-grade depression		Severe depression, suicide, other mental illness

until 14 years later did anyone ever confront him. **If you encounter behavior that troubles you, report it through established channels.**

Detecting and Healing Affective Blunting

Chapter 18 offers some generic strategies for emotional self-care. The "routine" and "taming the alter self" will help counteract diminished emotional responsiveness. Be alert for the appearance of your more insulated personality—the one you like least or that is most likely to "make" you feel guilty. Box 16.1 offers additional suggestions.

Activity: Repeatedly check your interactions with patients and colleagues. Try the following: While reading a write-up or recalling a patient encounter, ask yourself these questions:

- Was I open to the emotionally difficult parts of the patient's story?
- Did I "interrupt" the person when waiting or offering encouragement might have sparked him to continue?
- Did I feel emotional tension or pain? Did I shy away from it (e.g., asking a question that diverted the focus of the conversation)?
- Was I anxious to end the interview?
- Did I treat the patient (colleague) respectfully? Did he or she feel heard?

Formulate other questions to help increase your awareness.

The more often you monitor yourself, the more likely it will become habitual. Some people make it a part of their routine (see Chapter 18).

Notes

1. We are indebted to Eric Cassell (1991) for his clarifying work and writings on this subject. We have borrowed liberally from his thinking in this brief presentation and recommend his book.

2. This activity is adapted from Virshup, Bernard, M.D., in Coombs, Robert H., *Surviving Medical School,* Sage Publications, 1998. p. 30.

Part IV

Exiting the Clinical Years as a Whole and Well Person

17 Self-Care I

Personal Health Promotion and Medical Care

Health Promotion:
Exercise

How much happiness is gained and how much misery escaped, by frequent and violent agitation of the body.
                                                                    —Samuel Johnson

Exercise requires work, but it pays off in wellness. Healthy exercise can maintain and increase strength, provide flexibility, and improve aerobic stamina. It brings greater energy, more peaceful sleep, clears your mind, elevates mood, and like a safety valve, defuses the tensions of medical school. It may enhance the immune system and is salutary to bowel function. The right exercise will relax you and be enjoyable. If you already have a routine, do your best to maintain it during clerkships, but any exercise will be beneficial.

Aerobic Exercise

As medical students, you learn the parameters for effective aerobic exercise. Twenty to 30 minutes three to five times a week of brisk walking, running, roller blading, cycling, swimming, aerobic dance, or a comparable activity will maintain good aerobic conditioning. An aerobic workout should bring your heart rate into the target range (65-80% of 220 minus your age). Short warm-up and cool-down periods are always advised. Although not as refreshing as 20 to 30 continuous minutes, a few minutes of aerobic activity here and there during the day are cumulative. Hence, climbing stairs (avoiding the elevator), a walk at lunchtime, and parking your car away from your destination, are all valuable and feasible.

Flexibility

Stretching and hatha yoga maintain flexibility. For your frame—your musculoskeletal-fascial-joint system—this is vitally important. Brief stretches done in street clothes or scrubs at times during the day help a lot. You can assume certain yoga and stretching postures while on rounds or even in conferences. Many postures help release backlogs of emotional tension as well.

Strength

We do not advocate strenuous body building, but brief workouts two to four times a week with five to seven pound hand weights (or body-building machines) improve strength and posture and slow or prevent the appearance of osteoporosis. Push-ups and abdominal crunches are helpful as well.

Health Promotion:
Nutrition

> If doctors of today will not become the nutritionists of tomorrow, the nutritionists of today will become the doctors of tomorrow.
> —*Thomas Edison*

Psychology of Food

We must eat to survive. Food, our monogamous calorie source and companion for life, can be a source of much genuine and healthy pleasure. However, we also use it as a substitute for love and affection, as a salve for emotional pain, and to defuse anger. Thus, our commitment to it is often skewed in unhealthy ways. Avoidance of food (anorexia) and self-induced vomiting to disgorge food (bulimia) are not uncommon clinical problems, but 40% to 60% of

Americans are overweight. Nicotine dependence may help control appetite, but when the nicotine is stopped, weight gain is common. It can be "malignant" in magnitude.

> This was the case for Barnaby. Addicted to alcohol until the age of 32, he continued to smoke after becoming sober. Ten years later, he stopped tobacco and began gaining weight. He is now 70 pounds overweight, eats with awesome gluttony, and "wants to stop" but resists all help to do so. B's mother is morbidly obese, and his wife of 20 years shares his avarice for food and is obese. She, like Barnaby and his mother, has no desire to stop overeating.

Addictions to sugar and caffeine have patterns similar to drug addiction.

Principles for Healthy Eating

The following principles for healthy eating embody the thinking of most nutritional experts and health maintenance enthusiasts:

• Since no single food group contains all the nutrients you need, strive for variety in your food. This means selecting your food from all the major food groups: fresh and frozen fruits and vegetables; whole grains and grain products; dried peas, beans, and nuts; animal products—meat and dairy (limit intake of this last group except for very low-fat and no-fat products). Eating different foods also decreases the likelihood of exposure to harmful additives and toxins and helps restrict fat intake. The average American diet contains over 50% of calories as fat; 10% to 20% is probably the most effective level for preventing coronary atherosclerosis and heart attack.

• Use *unprocessed* (this term includes fresh frozen foods) and (in general) low-fat or nonfat foods. They provide more vitamins and minerals per unit volume and (in general) contain less saturated fat, free sugar, and salt, as well as fewer undesirable contaminants.

• Practice moderation—an old adage increasingly supported by modern science. It is particularly important in this regard that you drastically limit or avoid free sugar. Rising blood glucose levels stimulate insulin increase; rising insulin levels in turn increase appetite. This, of course, prevents insulin shock but, if repetitive, leads to overeating.

Table 17.1 Food Selection for Healthy Fare

Embrace (nutritious, low in calories)	Use as Required (nutritious but caloric)	Avoid/Use Rarely (unhealthy and very caloric)
Fresh vegetables and sprouts	Whole grain or lightly milled	Most fast foods (CND)[a]
Most frozen vegetables	bread and pasta	Many snack foods (CND)
Legumes: dried, canned (WS)[b]	Avocado	Highly salted and/or high-fat
Potatoes (white & sweet),	Honey	foods
corn, yams	Mayonnaise & salad	Most baked cakes and cookies
Veggie juices (WS)	dressings (WC)[c]	(CND)
Fresh and dried fruit (WC)[c]	No-salt nut butters	Lunchmeat and prepared
Cereals without sugar or salt	Soft margarine without	meats, organ meats
(puffed rice, Grapenuts,	trans-fatty acids	Full-fat dairy products
oatmeal) (CND)	Vegetable oils, especially	Candy
Fish,[d] fowl without skin	olive, except palm and	
	coconut	

NOTE: If your present diet is composed mostly of foods in the right-hand column, plan to change gradually—perhaps one major change every three to four months. Over a two-year period, this will result in significant alterations of your food intake toward a healthier pattern.

a. Check nutritional data.
b. Watch salt.
c. Watch calories.
d. Increasingly, fish of various kinds are being shown to contain heavy metals and agricultural toxins to a significant degree. This is most pronounced for fish from small lakes that drain artificially "enriched" soil.

- In certain physiological illness and stressful states (such as medical school and residency!), added care and restorative measures are indicated. Pregnancy, breast-feeding, sleep deprivation, any illness, and most dysfunctional stress situations are indications for careful attention to the first three principles as well as an enhanced intake of vitamins.

On a nutritional fare that has variety; is low in fat, sugar, and salt; and mostly avoids processed foods, you will feel healthier most of the time. Table 17.1 highlights the principles stated above and gives partial lists for very healthy, moderately healthy, and unhealthy foods.

Vitamin Supplements

A balanced diet containing sufficient fresh fruits and vegetables probably contains adequate vitamins. However, affordable fresh fruits and vegetables are not always available, and knowledge about degradation of naturally occurring vitamins during food processing, transportation, and storage is still primitive.

We advocate taking a multivitamin preparation, providing 100% of the RDI for each of the B complex vitamins, A, C, D, E, and folate. Additional vitamin C (up to 6 gm per day) is recommended by some for its antioxidant properties (to help prevent cancer) and for ameliorating and preventing upper-respiratory infections.

What About Being a Vegetarian?

Activity: Experiment with different amounts of dietary meat. Look for differences in your sense of well-being, moods, and energy levels.

Health Promotion:
Safety

Safety and accident prevention is a major concern for all health care workers. Medical students are in their 20s and 30s. In those age groups, accidents (mostly auto), homicide, suicide, and malignancy are leading causes of mortality. The serious illnesses are those transmitted by fecal contamination, respiratory droplets, and infected blood (Hepatitis B, AIDS). Anxiety and depression are also common. These issues, then, define your main concerns in terms of health and safety.

We advise the following:

- **Wash your hands frequently while at work,** certainly after examining a patient.

- **Wear a mask and wash your hands** when a serious condition can be transmitted by respiratory droplets. Although masks hinder rapport with patients, you can gain skill at relating from behind a mask. Masks are not foolproof. If a patient has pneumonia or another disease with respiratory transmission, politely ask him or her to avert his or her head while you do your exam or procedure. Patients seldom take this request personally.

- **Ask the head nurse or his or her surrogate to brief you on the protocols of the unit for drawing blood, doing arterial sticks, starting IVs and central lines, and other procedures where contact with the patient's blood is a risk. Do this on each clerkship.** Health care workers are accidentally stuck by needles 800,000 times a year; 12,000 of those will contract Hepatitis B (Turk, 1993).

- **Always wear seat belts in the car,** even if traveling only a short way. A colleague who elected not to use his seat belt for a five-block ride was hit by another car, thrown under a truck, and suffered compound fractures of both legs.

- **Designate a nondrinking driver or take a cab or bus home** if you have more than one alcoholic drink. If a friend is about to drive under the influence, ask for his or her key.

- **Practice safe sex.** With a new partner, any unprotected sex is risky until both of you have a negative HIV test drawn six months after sexual contact with others. Informed, intelligent, and otherwise responsible adults do not always heed this warning. If you're on the make, go prepared with condoms. The wisest course is to abstain from sex until you believe a relationship will have some durability.

- **Make sure your smoke alarm works.** Check it at least every six months, change the battery at the same time.

Health Promotion: Vacations and Time Off

Take all of the vacation and out-of-town meeting time to which you are entitled. The latter is seldom a problem, because for students there is rarely such entitlement. Vacation time is fixed between clerkships. Sometimes you have a choice between another elective and vacation time. Our recommendation is, take the time off, no matter what the elective. Staying sane during medical school (see "Subduing the 'Alter Self,' " Chapter 18) is not easy. *Time completely away from medical school is an antidote to exhaustion and dysfunctional stress.*

Time off is somewhat different. The discipline of patient care (Chapter 5) can require working beyond your assigned duty time. These are often fruitful hours. Do not by any means compromise all or most of your time off, but if an occasion suggests "extending yourself for the good of the patient" (Chapter 5) consider it. Sometimes, with a flexible house staff and attending, you will get time off in payback for the extra hours.

Medical Care for Yourself

Ideally, all medical students would participate in medical and health promotion programs designed explicitly for health professional trainees. Students could seek periodic health exams, help for illness, birth control, advice on the prevention of AIDS and other sexually transmitted disease, and good dental care. They could exercise in an easily accessible facility with well-maintained equipment and watch tapes on health maintenance. The school cafeteria would offer healthy, economical food and nutritional analyses. There is no better way to teach good medical care and the values of an effective health care system than by having trainees participate as patients and providers. Lamentably, only a handful of professional schools even begin to achieve this.

With no prior exposure to a good system, clerkship students too often treat themselves—with and without advice from residents and/or attendings. The dining room, scrub alcove, or hallway is the consulting venue for sick medical students. Sometimes a throat is examined; occasionally, a urinalysis or a hematocrit is done. The quick fix is practiced too often (Chapter 15). The pills come from someone's drawer or pocket—or from the omnipresent "drug rep." Schools may require you to carry health insurance, but few policies seem tailored to student needs.

Checklist for Personal Health and Illness Care

- Choose a primary care physician; meet with him or her and partner(s).
- Obtain copies of old health and medical records.
- Update immunization record.
- Review safety and health promotion measures.
- Update your health appraisal, including health questionnaire.
- Identify sources for medications as needed.
- Learn about health insurance.
- Find an exercise facility.
- Plan ahead for vacations and time *really off.*

If your school does not have a health program or does not designate a specific student health physician, find yourself a conveniently located primary care physician. See him or her before your first clerkship if possible. Take your immunization record and any other information you have about your medical history—old charts, hospital summary, results of lab tests. Discuss risks of the clerkships to which you are assigned, your immunization status, and how to avoid illness. Ask how to get a special appointment if there are no openings when you call. If he or she has a partner, ask to be introduced. Ask for advice about health insurance. (The dean for student affairs may also keep information on file.)

Activity: Fill out a questionnaire as part of your own health appraisal. If one is not available, ask the student health office or a primary care attending to provide you with one.

Make sure your physician creates a copy of your chart for you to keep. Keep it up to date and carry it with you from one move to the next. It will save you a lot of inconvenience and perhaps money.

Your personal health care system should model the system you want to provide for your patients. It should emphasize safety measures and health promotion and prevention as much as it does illness and injury care, and it should provide for emotional counseling and therapy as needed.

18 Self-Care II

Taking Care of Your Head, Heart, and Relationships

We don't need to burn out or burn up; we just need to keep burning on.
—*Anonymous*

This chapter addresses the prevention and care of emotional stress and personal depletion with particular attention to the wounds of the hidden (unstated) curriculum (Part III). We offer several strategies for maintaining emotional/spiritual health: the "routine," controlling the alter self, healthy attitudes, adequate rest, patience, emotional support, asking for help, and living in day-tight compartments. Further strategies specific to affective blunting and loss of intellectual vitality are in the self-care boxes of Chapters 15 and 16. This chapter also speaks to preserving relationships. Other books in this series will cover self-care and relationships in greater detail.

Generic Strategies for Emotional Health

The "Routine"

Most emotionally healthy people living reasonably balanced, effective lives have multidimensional health promotion routines. *They do certain things daily and others regularly one or two times a week:*[1] for example, exercise, yoga or stretching, reading, listening to or making music, time with family, gardening, time in nature, spiritual practices (reading, prayer, meditation, affirmations, yoga again), and emotional support (talking regularly to partner, counselor, support group). Most routines include two or more of these foundational activities and otherwise vary widely to include ordinary activities such as taking vitamins, brushing and flossing teeth, walking the dog, listening to the news, or going to church.

When you omit the ordinary activities, it's like a blinking yellow light—proceed with caution. Having neglected flossing for two days, you are warned to review the rest of your routine. If you neglect one of your foundational activities (like talking to someone on a regular basis), it's a red light. You need to take a look at your whole process. *An explicit routine gives your life trustworthy and compelling order. It is the core of health maintenance.*

Be aware when your routine is slipping. It is fine to change it, but do so consciously, not by defaulting a foundational aspect.

Sample Routine for a Medical Student

- Walk to work
- Attend morning report
- Weekly handball game
- Run 3 times weekly
- Brush teeth, bid; floss, qd
- Two hands of cards qw
- An apple a day
- Daily inspirational reading
- Take vitamins

Activity: Identify the most important activities in your routine and decide how you will continue them during clerkships perhaps on a reduced time basis.

Subduing the "Alter Self"

In a sense, the concept of "dual personality" applies to most of us. Our usual personality gets the work done, coexists with others, and is more accessible emotionally and intellectually. The "alter self" is isolative, argumentative, self-pitying, and behaves badly. It may also be grumpy, self-critical, and defensive. For some individuals, the two personalities can be quite different, for others, only subtly so.

Resisting ascension of the alter self is a second generic strategy for taking care of yourself. Usually, we live in our more effective role, but the alter self is adept at ambush and disguise. When aware of its presence, some people are good at hiding it. Others deny its presence. However, by acknowledging the reality of the second personality, we learn to tell when it is present or about to appear. We can deal with it more effectively.

Samantha was 27 and a medical school junior. After college, she was in the Peace Corps for two years, then ran a social rehab program for the homeless. Her references for medical school spoke glowingly of her competence and emotional sensitivity. Devoted to her church, she facilitated a support group to help teenagers deal with the pressures to smoke, drink, and be sexually involved. She resigned that responsibility halfway through second year due to academic pressure. After four weeks on her clerkship in internal medicine, the patient advocate notified the clerkship coordinator that three patients had filed complaints against Samantha: "She was abrupt," "didn't listen closely," and/or "didn't seem to like me"—all in sharp contrast to her previous evaluations. Hearing these complaints, Samantha sobbed, "This is terrible. I am exhausted, not sleeping well, and I dream about injuring my patients. This clerkship has been so hard. I don't understand it. In the Peace Corps we lived primitively, worked long hours, and saw a lot of squalor and sickness, but this is much more difficult." The clerkship coordinator learned that Samantha had blotted out the rest of her life "to do a good job on the clerkship." She spent hours during her time "off" keeping up with scut work and charting. She stopped exercising, attending church, and visiting friends and family. An enlightened coordinator gave her a week off without penalty and urged her to seek counseling and form a support group. During the rest of the clerkship, Samantha participated regularly in the support group and was her "old self." Her nightmares disappeared, and her sleeping normalized. Patients were delighted with her.

Samantha had regressed into an alter self that affected her work with patients. It was quiescent for years when she had regular emotional and spiritual support.

Healthy Attitudes

Examine your attitudes toward work. Both the explicit and unstated curricula affect them. Watch out especially for cynicism and resentments. A clerkship can always be better: more teaching, fewer nights on call, more procedures, and greater diversity of patients. But medical schools are administratively and politically complex, so the likelihood of reassignment or significant change is slim. Don't hesitate to suggest worthwhile changes in teaching sessions, but be ready to accept things as they are. Remember that *you are the principal variable in how much you learn.* The healthy attitude is, "Though it is not ideal, I choose to make the most of this clerkship." Be ready to get the work done on time and without grousing—at least not in earshot of your teachers!

Activity: With your faculty members and other students, set priorities for your work and clarify uncertainties and concerns. What takes priority—rounds or new admissions? Do we (the students) select cases for neurology conference? Find out what's essential, what's not.

Adequate Rest

Reserve time for yourself on a regular basis. This includes taking your nights off . . . really off and catching up with sleep.

Emotional Support

Bad dreams, intrusive daytime fantasies, and/or the alter self may appear during clerkships. You will experience emotionally trying episodes. Talk about them to a partner, close friend, or mentor in whom you can confide safely. A support group that meets every two weeks or so is an excellent way of talking to colleagues. If none exists, form one. A faculty person or group members can facilitate it in turn.

Spiritual Enrichment

If you have a spiritual program, stay with it (see Chapter 19). Have fun; this advice sounds trivial, but it is not. Fun is fuel for the spirit. Find time, even if only five minutes a day, for a hobby or pastime you enjoy.

Be Patient

On the virtue, patience, J. Ruth Gendler (1984) writes, "You don't notice her right away in a crowd, but suddenly you see her all at once, and then she is so beautiful you wonder why you never saw her before" (p. 5).

Asking for Help

Many of us staunchly resist asking for help. We deny that we need it, or we ask for it too late. **Ask for help**—with your patients, with other work, with important decisions and or preoccupations. For example, if your roster of patients gets too large, transfer a patient to your colleagues.

Live in Day-Tight Compartments

Live as deeply as possible in the present. Your next patient may switch you on. Dr. William Carlos Williams tells of being totally exhausted after a long day's work, only to be completely reenergized by an unexpected patient late in the day. Goethe said, "Nothing is worth more than this day." Include exercise, relaxation, or amusement as part of your day-tight compartments (Osler, 1932b).

Specific Steps for
Managing Emotional Unresponsiveness
(Affective Blunting)

Affective blunting is common in medical school and clerkships (Chapter 16). For years, such emotional detachment was considered essential to practice medicine. "Pure objectivity" was the basis of good decisions. Indeed, it can deter your own needs from taking precedence over the patients', but this can be achieved in healthier ways. Your authors believe that the best decisions are guided to varying degrees by an intuition fine-tuned by appropriate emotional vulnerability.

Of greater importance, detachment shields you from the emotional issues of your patients and from your own emotional reactions. Many patient complaints about physician rapport (and sometimes performance) are stimulated by physician impassivity. For these reasons, the processing and resolution of feelings aroused by events in patient care is extremely important. Unprocessed, they will sap your energy and spirit and change your personality and lifestyle in ways that are inimical to the best practice of medicine.

In addition to the generic strategies discussed in the preceding section, several specific ones to help prevent or counteract affective blunting are given in the self-care box of Chapter 16 (p. 157).

Specific Suggestions for
Averting Intellectual Stagnation

Although Chapter 15 is foreboding, a further decline of intellectual vitality during clerkships can, with attention and diligence, be arrested or reversed. The generic strategies outlined above (pp. 172-175) for preserving emotional health and responsiveness can also preserve your intellectual vitality. Further suggestions are given in the self-care box of Chapter 15 (p. 147).

Relationships: Double Meanings

Healthy, close human relationships are the *sine qua non* of personal support and nurture—nothing is more essential. Despite this, "[Just as] the impact of abrupt status change and adaptation to stress are left to the individual student . . . , so is the adjustment to alienation from family, friends, and the outside world" (Coombs, 1998, p. 5).

Nevertheless, students know that their morale and emotional health in medical school can benefit greatly from strong relationships; spouse or partner relationships and friendships were mentioned most frequently. One student said, "[There] has to be somebody for emotional support. . . . little things make a difference . . . knowing there will be someone else there [is important]." Third-year students involved in a stable primary relationship attributed major importance to it in "getting me through." "I have a good support system in my girlfriend and can relate to her about most emotional problems." Families of origin were not always helpful. "My parents aren't helpful—they don't understand the system."

Paradoxically, while affirming the support of good relationships, many students we interviewed lamented diminution or failure of their own. *In the face of medical school pressures, important relationships are at great risk.* Students often choose to terminate or weaken them. Several new third-year students had recently ended a partner relationship or were avoiding serious relationships, seeing them as a hindrance to successful passage through medical school and residency. One student ended a close three-year relationship midway through first year because "becoming a good physician has highest priority. I don't see this as healthy—only as a necessary choice."

Sadly, medical school administrators, faculty members, and the culture are appreciably indifferent to the fate of students' personal relationships. They support the unbalanced work ethic of medical training and state or imply that the demands of medical school should discourage high priorities on anything but "medicine." Even marriages and partnerships between two medical students are powerfully stressed.

> I think before I came to medical school I wondered why so many of the marriages broke up, and now I think I know why. . . . For me, it's been very stressful. I've done a lot of crying the last few years. Both of us were at very stressful points in our lives. I can't imagine what it would be like to do this with children. Both of us felt like we needed a wife, mother, and housekeeper—all rolled into one. Neither of us had the energy to be that with the other person.

When relationships ended, students grieved privately if at all. Few took advantage of support groups or counseling services even if these resources were available. *No student reported having a counseling or supportive relationship with a faculty member.* If one of your family members or an important friend suffers illness or dies, the meaningfulness of the underlying relationship and the importance of your loss may not be acknowledged through administrative flexibility or personal offers of support from faculty or administrators. We have never seen an examination waived because of such occurrences. One woman missed a week of clerkship following her mother's death. She was required to repeat the entire 12-week clerkship—a pejorative sentence in response to a grievous personal loss. Students involved in such unfortunate circumstances remained well behaved and in effect condoned the institutional indifference. Fearing some administrative "retaliation" or a penalizing grade, they did not expect or ask for special considerations. They took little or no time away from school.

Implications for
Your Future Relationships With Patients

Consumers of medical care lament that the model physician-patient relationship is not as empathetic, caring, and collaborative as they would like. We believe the precariousness of medical students' own personal relationships and the flimsy relationships between medical schools and their students are major roots of these failings.

Like close personal relationships, strong, helpful relationships with your patients require commitment and attention. *The physician who builds meaningful relationships with patients is, in all likelihood, one who consistently honors his or her relationships with friends and family.* Although the importance of healthy doctor-patient relationships is trumpeted by medical educators and institutions, these same institutions treat their students like objects. The importance of "honoring the student" is not acknowledged by institutions and/or the departments that sponsor clerkships. The implied message from the schools and departments is that relationships are not important. Therefore, you must be vigilant. This institutional shortcoming can seriously dilute good intentions on your part to make *relationship* the center of your care for patients.

Activity: What is your history with partnering relationships? How long have they lasted? How do they end? What has been difficult for you? Have you made lasting friendships? How many lasting friendships (more than five years duration, see in person one or more times a year, talk to every month or two) have you had since age 14?

Maintaining and Nourishing Important Relationships

You should not sacrifice or seriously wound important personal relationships on the altar of medical education. Doing so is contradictory to learning how to relate to patients in a committed way and deprives you of important sources of support. Here are some suggested stratagems for maintaining and nourishing important relationships:

- **Be realistic; warn people ahead of time.** Before the year begins, tell your important people that there will be periods when you will not be able to give them as much time as you would like.

- **Select two or three most important relationships (MIRs). Recommit to them.** Be assertive; ask them to go more than half way, knowing you can reciprocate in the future. After a month or two, discuss how the plan is working; honesty is of the essence.

- **Be available to each MIR at least twice a month: a phone call, a visit—even if brief—or a meal together. Stick by these commitments; it will pay off.**

Activity: Reread the material on interviewing/listening in Chapter 9. Apply those basic rules to your personal relationships.

- **Every 10 to 14 days, spend 10 to 15 minutes talking to an MIR about the clerkship. If you are macho (or macha!), you may find this hard. But it's important. Just talking about traumatic or stressful events is salutary.**

- **Don't make drastic changes in relationships during a clerkship.** Don't end or significantly change friendships or partnerships (although the other party may not give you any choice). Avoid intense new relationships. A liaison begun during a busy clerkship can be heady. It will also be fragile. The combination can lead to a lot of pain.

- **Acknowledge important family times by phone or in person**—certain major holidays, birthdays, and religious observances. Rituals are important in preventing substance abuse and other unhealthy behaviors. In addition to spiritual or religious ones, rituals might include a weekly dinner together, a TV show, attendance at a young person's athletic or artistic events, regular trips to the library.

A Final Word

The effort necessary to maintain strong relationships while negotiating medical school (and residency) often feels impossible to mobilize. When directed at the right people, it invariably turns out to be worth it.

Activity:

1. In five minutes, describe to a friend one initially strong relationship that went sour. Then describe (five minutes) a relationship with a patient that was difficult or ended on a disturbing note. Are there any parallels or sharp contrasts?

2. Select one or two stratagems that might help you stay in committed relationships.

Note

1. Of course, one can have a destructive routine—for example, the addict who must have his line of cocaine before starting the day or the obsessive-compulsive who must mop and scrub the bathroom and kitchen daily before anything else gets done.

19 Spirituality

The Quiet Answer

Listen to your life. See it for the fathomless mystery that it is. In the boredom and pain of it no less than in the excitement and gladness: touch, taste, smell your way to the holy and hidden heart of it because in the last analysis all moments are key moments, and life itself is grace.
—*Frederick Buechner (1983, p. 92)*

Although we favor an openness to the contributions of spiritual experience and practice for modern medicine, we also want to acknowledge a deep historical difficulty. Throughout history, people's beliefs or nonbeliefs about God have been used to segregate, relocate, and persecute them. This has led, in some quarters, to an understandable resistance to the spiritual. Such hesitations are honestly felt and need to be respected. We speak of spirituality here as a dimension that is common across all people—"inclusive spirituality" (Thomason & Brody, 1999). We deplore any use of the spiritual that divides people or creates hierarchy. *In acknowledging a spiritual dimension of medicine, we do not proselytize for any particular church or body of faith.*

Clarification of Terms

Your *spirituality* manifests the best of yourself. It expresses the values and meanings without which you will founder. It involves the acquisition, expres-

181

sion, and honoring of those qualities, values, and behaviors that define the kind of person you want to be. It is, for most of us, the essence of our bond to other individuals, to family, to larger communities of friendship and service, and to a transcendent being or set of values. To be religious, by contrast, requires significant adherence to, and/or membership in, a specific organized or institutionalized body of faith—Buddhism, Catholicism, Judaism.

Among those who characterize themselves as spiritual rather than religious, many do, nevertheless, draw parts of their spirituality from the teachings and practices of one or more religions. Others in the spiritual group are deeply spiritual without being at all religious. Among those who consider themselves religious, most, to varying degrees, see their spirituality sustained by other elements as well as by their chosen body of faith. Rarely, an individual will say he or she is religious and "not spiritual," and for a few, their religion "is (in toto) my spirituality."

Thomason and Brody (1999) cite Rachel Naomi Remen, MD, who "suggests that the spiritual is that realm of human experience to which religion attempts to connect us (sometimes successfully, sometimes not) through doctrine, ritual, and practice. 'Religion is a bridge to the spiritual but the spiritual lies beyond religion' " (p. 96).

Activity: Describe your own spirituality to a friend. What activities can you do every day to nurture and stimulate your spiritual self?

Why Acknowledge a Spiritual Dimension to Medicine?

We accept spirituality as an essential dimension of medical education and practice for the following reasons.

• Even if you do not follow a specific religion or consider yourself a spiritual being, a majority of your patients will be "spiritual," and most will believe in God, a higher power, or a universal energy (i.e., a transcendental being). Thus, Lebacqz (1986), echoed by Foglio and Brody (1988), states that physicians who wish to heal must confront the variables of faith, religion, and spirituality, because whether recognized or not, they operate in the patient-physician transaction.

- Many patients want their physicians to pay more attention to the spiritual dimension (Daaleman & Nease, 1994).

- Many patients believe that religious and other spiritual practices can enhance healing. Bringing one's spiritual beliefs and practices to bear on one's illness assists resolution and provides a source of hope.[1] For over 50 years, Alcoholics Anonymous and other 12-step programs have demonstrated how an inclusive spiritual program is capable of healing addictive illnesses—an area in which conventional medicine has enjoyed little or no success.

- A number of medical schools now offer courses for medical students on spirituality and medicine. Two of your authors helped plan and implement one of them.[2] The students have enthusiastically received it. They see that it is acceptable and feasible to inquire about spiritual beliefs and practices and to help patients use their own spirituality to aid healing. Many students say the course stimulated them to enrich their own spiritual lives and to be more attentive to personal well-being.

Spirituality, Religion, and Medicine

So the relationship between one's religion and one's spirituality can be simple—there is usually some confluence—and complex, in that it is different for almost everyone. *An individual's spiritual beliefs and practices are almost always felt as supportive, whereas his or her religious ties may not be.*

The implications for the spiritual dimension of medicine are clear. In Figure 19.1, all drawings depict an individual whose spirituality and religion overlap. *Medicine* signifies an individual's health promotion practices, an illness, an injury, or a rehabilitation effort. The left-hand diagram shows that the individual's health promotion program draws to a significant degree on her spirituality. In the middle drawing, she has an attack of migraine (Illness A) that is treated and subsides within 12 hours. She misses only one day of work. No explicit additional spiritual activity is stimulated by the episode. The right-hand diagram depicts the same individual suffering the discovery of colon cancer (Illness B), its subsequent removal, and a prolonged convalescence. Uncer-

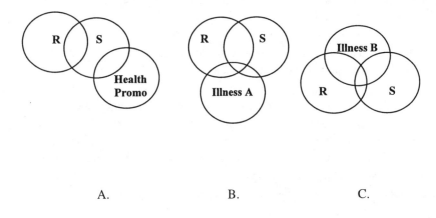

A.   B.   C.

Figure 19.1. Spirituality, Religion, and Medicine

tainty about metastases and prolonged absence from work resulted in an extended illness. The patient was fearful, uncertain, and modified her lifestyle to include regular prayer and meditation. "God's help and blessings" were solicited by the patient and her family on many occasions both in church services and at other times. Clearly, the spiritual dimension of her illness received considerable attention.

Suggestions for Exploring the Spiritual Dimension With Patients

- Be comfortable with your own spirituality.
- Consider the suggested spiritual perspectives in Box 19.1. Try manifesting some or all of them.
- Gain trust by using terminology acceptable to the patient (for some patients *God* is not the right word) and by using appropriate and careful self-disclosure about your spirituality. **Do not proselytize.**
- Explore the patient's spirituality with subsets of the questions in Box 19.2. There are many others that could be used as well. "Give permission" for the patient to

---

BOX 19.1

**Suggested Spiritual Perspectives
for Caregivers**

- It is a privilege to learn my patients' stories, including the intimate details of their lives.
- It is a privilege to share responsibility for my patients' well-being.
- Patients must make their own choices; I can only influence and advise.
- Many outcomes are greatly influenced by variables over which I have no control; I am often powerless over outcomes.
- Every human interaction is either an act of love or a cry for help.
- One can be quite spiritual without belonging to a church or adhering to a specific body of faith.
- Death is not an enemy; it is a spiritual transition.
- I do not always know what's going on when it's going on (in the larger sense).

---

dwell on his or her spiritual world. With respect to spirituality, we can never know everything to ask, but many of the suggested queries will help people reveal their own unique spirituality.

Red Lights and Reservations

To some patients (and faculty members), pursuing the spiritual dimension may seem too time-consuming, uncomfortable, contrived, or inappropriate. **If a patient seems uncomfortable discussing spiritual issues, the best course may be to refrain.** Subsequently, formal or informal assistance from a pastoral counselor or chaplain may be fruitful. **Also, it is hazardous and inappropriate to pursue the spiritual dimension in a proselytizing spirit.** Some caregivers emphasize the spiritual focus to the detriment of thorough diagnosis and management.

BOX 19.2

Exploring Your Patients' Spirituality

- What was your religious background, upbringing, or faith as a child?
- Do you still hold and practice those beliefs?
- What or who gives particular meaning or strength to your life?
- Where do you turn in times of desperation?
- Are your spirituality and religion different?
- Is religion or God important to you now?
- Do you attend any group activities that are religious or spiritual (including church)?
- Do you pray, meditate, or "exercise your spirit" in other ways?
- What effect may your illness have on your spiritual practices or beliefs and vice versa?
- How can we help you maintain your spiritual strength?
- Can your spiritual beliefs and practices help prevent or minimize illness in the future?
- Do you believe in God, some higher power, or a universal force or energy?
- Is there anything else you want me to know about your beliefs?

Other Barriers to Integrating a Spiritual Dimension Into Your Work With Patients

- Your peers, supervisors, and/or teachers may downplay, ignore, or disagree with exploring spirituality as an integral part of the care process.
- Many services engage in crisis-directed, reactive care. Involvement in the spiritual dimension is more proactive. Clinical busyness focuses on diagnosis and curing. Healing is not widely acknowledged as a different concept from curing (see glossary).
- Patient resistance. On rare occasions, the patient may see exploration of the spiritual dimension as taking time from the real business of diagnosis and curing—the quick fix.

Nurturing Your Own Spirituality

After many years in academic medicine, Lee, M.D., elected to do urgent care with a large HMO. Each shift, he saw four to five patients an hour for 8 to 10 hours. Patient's problems varied from colds to heart attacks, some requiring lab work, X-rays, or both. It was hectic work. Lee commonly fell behind schedule and feared that he'd miss something or give patients inadequate attention. In the fifth week, one morning was particularly arduous. Three extra patients were scheduled, and there were several diagnostic problems. Lee felt tight, inadequate, and rushed. He was "brusque with at least two patients that morning." At 10:30, he still had nine patients to see before noon. Picking up the chart for his next patient, Lee grasped the doorknob of the examining room, took a deep breath and was "compelled to whisper, 'God please help me do my best in here.' " The ensuing encounter was relaxed and efficient. Both Lee and his patient left feeling satisfied and peaceful. From then on, "mystified but encouraged," Lee said a short prayer before meeting each patient. He worked in urgent care another 14 months, which he found "totally satisfying and relatively nonstressful."

Whatever you do with patients, we encourage you to attend to your own spirituality and values clarification. We perceive that students and physicians with explicit spiritual beliefs and practices derive significant comfort and support from them. For example, spiritual work helps people cope with sad, traumatic, repulsive, and anger-provoking situations involving loved ones, patients, colleagues, teachers, and managed care. Other benefits include the following:

- Exploring a patient's spirituality when you are fostering your own often imparts a peacefulness to the relationship not easily found in other ways.
- "Being with the patient" (Chapter 16) is facilitated by an alliance acknowledging spiritual practices, beliefs, and wisdom.

Suggested Strategies

- *Acknowledge that spiritual self-care requires regular spiritual practices just as physical fitness requires regular exercise.* Nourish your spirit daily in ways that work for you: music, dance, basketball, yoga, reading, meditation, prayer, affirmations.

- Respect your patients' and colleagues' spirituality.
- Communicate with patients about their spirituality when it is appropriate. Encourage them to bring it to bear on their illness. Providing such support and encouragement will nurture your spirit.
- Every one or two months, with a partner or friend, take a day for a seminar, a silent retreat, a visit with nature, or another activity that feels spiritually enriching to you.
- If you practice a particular religion or faith, continue as you are able. Go to services in your church/temple/mosque if they appeal to you. For many, the music alone is helpful.
- Learn to quiet yourself with meditation, deep breathing, music, prayer, nature, time off.
- Playing or having fun (read, *pleasure*) is often a spirited or spirit-filled activity. Fun is a basic food group of spirituality—perhaps the fresh fruit. Healthy spirituality is possible without fun (unlike intention, the *essential protein* of spirituality), but you would miss a lot of pleasure. Play as you can; work when you must.
- If you have a spiritual adviser or counselor, use that person. If you don't, consider finding one. Remember that spiritual and emotional energy are closely related.

Activity:

1. Observe yourself for a week; note the essential icons, beliefs, affirmations, and other practices that fuel and renew your spirit.
2. Choose two or three of these activities that are feasible during clerkships. Plan to accomplish one or two of them each day.

Notes

1. Thus, spiritual or religious practices—prayer and meditation have been studied more thoroughly than others—can favorably influence the course of disease and illness and reduce suffering. For example, anonymous prayer for people on a coronary care unit increased short-term survival rates over those for whom no prayers were offered (Byrd, 1988).

2. This course has been given at Northeast Ohio Universities College of Medicine for three years. Lura Pethtel, dean of academic and student affairs participated in the planning and has been the administrator and one of two principal faculty members for the course since its inception.

Glossary

Affective blunting: See **diminished emotional responsiveness.**

Attending physician: The physician with ultimate responsibility for patients. The attending serves for two to eight weeks at a time, conducts rounds with house staff and/or students, and is generally available for advice 24 hours a day. In some hospitals, patients may have different attendings, each responsible for their own patients.

Circadian rhythms: Periodic biological cycles recurring at about 24-hour intervals.

Code: A euphemism for an urgent cardiac or respiratory emergency that threatens life. It is frequently used as part of the announcement or signal for such an emergency, as in "code blue." The verb form is also employed, as in "we coded the patient."

CPR (cardiopulmonary resuscitation): The procedures used to resuscitate the patient who has undergone cardiac or respiratory arrest. "We did CPR."

Critical questions: Questions that serve to advance or improve the care of a particular patient (Is there a potentially better way to protect this patient's immunologic capability than what we're doing now?) or to suggest an approach that might advance our knowledge of the patient's disease or a related problem (How might one develop evidence to support the hypothesis that this is primarily an infectious disorder rather than a degenerative one?).

Curing: The resolution or elimination of disease. "Her strep throat was cured."

Disease: A disorder or abnormality in structure or function of an organ or an organ system.

Diminished emotional responsiveness (DER) (also affective blunting): An impaired or severely restricted ability to feel one's own anger, sadness, fear, anxiety, and other emotional pain, and/or to deal with these feelings in ways that are healthy. Those who "stuff" their emotions are a common example. Commonly, among caregivers,

189

DER includes decreased or absent capability to acknowledge, be open to, and work effectively with the emotional and spiritual needs and reactions of one's patients.

DNR (do not resuscitate):   An alternate designation for the "no-code" patient.

Healing: Amelioration or resolution of an *illness* or the effects of an illness on the patient. The word may be used in reference to quite specific and tangible manifestations, as in "her wound has healed well," or it may be used to mean transition to a state of acceptance and greater peace in the face of prolonged illness or impending death. In *Healers on healing,* Carlson and Shield (1989) say, "Without love, there can be no true healing. For healing means not only a body without disease or injury, but a sense of forgiveness, belonging, and caring as well" (p. 3).

Illness: A broadened perspective of a pathological condition, disease, or sickness that encompasses the *impact* (effects) on the patient's personal life, job, family, friends, and at times, even the larger community (as when an individual's mental condition results in harm to others in the community or when one has a readily communicable disease). Illness also includes any *roots* of the sickness or pathology in the patient's personality, family dynamics, social status, or ethnic background. The patient's suffering and that of family and other loved ones is also part of illness.

Implicit curriculum: Highly significant aspects of almost every clerkship experience that most students do not anticipate and that often seem unrecognized by faculty as the highly formative phenomena they are. They include (a) the almost inevitable sad and draining aspects of patient care inevitably experienced in almost every clerkship; (b) certain teaching and evaluation strategies that demean, objectify, and often isolate students, and although not inevitable, are all too common; and (c) certain aspects of the environment. It is also referred to in this book as the unstated curriculum and the hidden curriculum.

Intellectual vitality: A state of robust and flexible intellectual activity with the salient traits of curiosity, creativity, the capability for divergent thinking, integrative capacity, medical problem solving, and tolerance for ambiguity. In medicine, intellectual vitality also includes a practical understanding of research methods.

Impairment: Physician impairment can range widely from simple inattention and carelessness to poorly managed anger and drug dependence (see Table 16.1).

Medical education: A term used to include the four years of medical school, residency training, and continuing education for practicing physicians.

MRI (magnetic resonance imaging)   A technique that provides more sophisticated, more detailed X-ray-like images used for diagnostic purposes.

No-code: The status of an individual patient for whom the decision has been made (by the patient himself or herself, relatives, or loved ones) to not do CPR if the patient stops breathing or has a cardiac arrest.

Premedical education: Usually the four years of college prior to entering medical school. For those who enter abbreviated (six-year) programs, the two years prior to entering medical school.

Rounds: In this book, rounds are sequential discussions about, and/or visitations paid to patients by the physicians and students responsible for their care.

Scut work: The work, sometimes considered demeaning, of performing essential tasks in patient care that may be simple and repetitive and that often seem uninteresting. Common ones include drawing blood for lab work; transporting blood, urine samples, and cultures to the lab; passing tubes of various kinds; doing throat and wound cultures; and starting IVs. Many of these tasks are exciting when you have never done them before but may feel boring and repetitive after you have done a few.

Service: The term is sometimes used in a way that is synonymous with *unit,* but more usually it denotes an entire specialty or subspecialty department, including the venues (in- and outpatient) in which patient care is delivered and the administrative and research areas as well. (If you are told the medical service is on the fourth floor, it usually means that both the patient care units and the administrative offices are there.)

Suffering: To endure pain, death, *or some other discomfort or distress.* In this realistically more complex view of suffering, distress often includes *that associated with events that threaten the intactness of the person.* Suffering, then, is predominately subjective on the part of the patient; it is wrapped in the meaning that patients' give to their illness or injury, and it can be completely known only through careful inquiry.

Teaching hospital: In the broadest sense, any hospital in which training of students and house staff occurs. A more insular meaning would insist that a teaching hospital is a university hospital or a closely and legally affiliated (for teaching purposes) hospital (such as the county hospital or the Veterans Administration) that trains large numbers of that university's students and residents.

Unit: A term used to indicate a geographically distinct set of rooms and spaces for the care of patients belonging to a particular specialty or subspecialty ("the cardiac unit"). Most clerkship assignments are to one such unit, although occasionally they involve more than one (e.g., in fourth year, your clerkship on nephrology might center on the inpatient renal unit but involve two half-days a week in the renal outpatient or follow-up clinic).

Abbreviations Used in This book

CPR—cardiorespiratory resuscitation (see glossary)
CSF—cerebrospinal fluid
DC—discontinue
DNR—do not resuscitate (see glossary)
H&P—history and physical exam
HCD—high-caloric density
LCD—low-caloric density
MAP—major active problem
MCD—medium-caloric density
MI—myocardial infarction (heart attack)
MRI—magnetic resonance imaging (see glossary)
MSW—medical social worker
NP—nurse practitioner
PA—physician's assistant
PCCC—primary care continuity clerkship
PE—physical exam
URI—upper-respiratory infection

References

Association of American Medical Colleges. (1982). *Survey for the general professional education of the physician and college preparation for medicine.* Washington, DC: Author.

Becker, E. (1973). *The denial of death.* New York: Free Press/Macmillan.

Bird, B. (1955). *Talking with patients.* Philadelphia, PA: Lippincott.

Bolton, R. (1979). *People skills.* New York, NY: Simon & Schuster.

Buber, M. (1958). *I and thou.* New York: Scribners.

Buechner, F. (1983). *Now and then.* New York: Harper & Row.

Burack, R. C., & Carpenter, R. (1983). The predictive value of the presenting complaint. *Journal of Family Practice, 16,* 749-754.

Byrd, R. (1988). Positive therapeutic effects of intercessory prayer in a coronary care unit population. *Southern Medical Journal, 81,* 826-829.

Carlson, R., & Shield, B. (1989). *Healers on healing.* New York: Tarcher/Putnam.

Cassell, E. J. (1976). *The healer's art.* New York: Penguin.

Cassell, E. J. (1991). *The nature of suffering and the goals of medicine.* New York: Oxford.

Coombs, R. H. (1998). *Surviving medical school.* Thousand Oaks, CA: Sage.

Covey, S. R. (1989). *The seven habits of highly effective people.* New York: Simon & Schuster.

Daaleman, P. P., & Nease, D. F. (1994). Patient attitudes regarding physician inquiry into spiritual and religious issues. *Journal of Family Practice, 39,* 564-568.

Enelow, A. J., & Swisher, S. N. (1972). *Interviewing and patient care.* New York: Oxford.

Enelow, A. J., Forde, D., & Brummel-Smith, K. (1996). *Interviewing and patient care* (4th ed.). New York: Oxford.

Finkelstein, P. (1986). Studies in the anatomy laboratory: A portrait of individual and collective defense. In R. H. Coombs, D. S. May, & G. W. Small (Eds.), *Inside doctoring: Stages and outcomes in the professional development of physicians* (pp. 22-42). New York: Praeger.

Foglio, J. P., & Brody, H. (1988). Religion, faith, and family medicine [editorial]. *Journal of Family Practice, 27,* 473-474.

Gendler, J. R. (1984). *The book of qualities.* Berkeley, CA: Turquoise Mountain.

Gusky, J. (1982). *Medical student ward survival manual.* Dallas, TX: Medical Student Publishers.

Hilfiker, R. (1991). Mistakes. In R. Reynolds & J. Stone (Eds.), *On doctoring* (pp. 376-387). New York: Simon & Schuster.

Lebacqz, K. (1986). Faith dimensions in medical practice. *Primary Care, 13,* 269.

Lederman, R. J. (1995). *How to be a truly excellent junior medical student.* Alexandria, VA: International Medical Publishing.

Levertov, D. (1991). Death psalm. In R. Reynolds & J. Stone (Eds.), *On doctoring* (pp. 257-258). New York: Simon & Schuster.

Lief, H. I., & Fox, R. C. (1963). Training for "detached concern" in medical students. In H. I. Lief, V. Lief, & N. R. Lief (Eds.,), *The psychological basis of medical practice* (pp. 12-35). New York: Hoeber/Harper & Row.

Lindbergh, A. M. (1955). *Gift from the sea.* New York: Pantheon.

Lowenstein, J. (1997). *The midnight meal and other essays.* New Haven, CT: Yale.

Marion, R. (1991). *Learning to play God.* New York: Fawcett Crest.

Osler, W. (1932a). *Aequanimitas with other addresses.* New York: Blakiston.

Osler, W. (1932b). *A way of life.* Baltimore, MD: Remington-Putnam.

Osler, W. (1995). Aphorisms. In R. Reynolds & J. Stone (Eds.), *On doctoring* (2nd ed., pp. 30-33). New York: Simon & Schuster.

Paget, M. A. (1988). *The unity of mistakes.* Philadelphia, PA: Temple.

Peck, M. S. (1978).*The road less traveled.* New York: Simon & Schuster.

Peterson, M. C., Holbrook, J. H., Van Hales, M. D., et al. (1992). Contributions of the history, physical examination, and laboratory investigation in making medical diagnoses. *Western Journal of Medicine, 156,* 163-165.

Polk, R. (1995). *The medical student's survival guide* (4th ed.). Myrtle Beach, SC: MedEnCom/Treatland.

Reynolds, R., & Stone, J. (1991). *On doctoring.* New York: Simon & Schuster.

Reynolds, R. & Stone, J. (1995). *On doctoring* (revised and expanded). New York: Simon & Schuster.

Stone, J. (1991). Gaudeamus igitur. In R. Reynolds & J. Stone (Eds.), *On doctoring* (pp. 347-351). New York: Simon & Schuster.

Thomason, C. L., & Brody, H. (1999). Inclusive spirituality [editorial]. *Journal of Family Practice, 48*(2), 96-97.

Turk, M. (1993, September). High anxiety. *The new physician,* pp. 16-22.

Ways, P. O. (1985). *Take charge of your health.* Lexington, MA: Stephen Greene.

Whitehead, A. N. (1957). *The aims of education and other essays.* New York: Free Press/Macmillan. (Original work published in 1929)

Williams, W. C. (1991). The practice. In R. Reynolds & J. Stone (Eds.), *On doctoring* (pp. 72-77). New York: Simon & Schuster.

Worby, C. (1972). Interviewing the family. In A. Enelow & S. Swisher (Eds.), *Interviewing and patient care.* New York: Oxford.

Index

About the Authors

Dr. Peter Ways has taught students in all four years of medical school—as a lecturer and group leader in biochemistry and laboratory science, and in clinical medicine as an internist and hematologist. At Michigan State University's College of Human Medicine, he devoted himself entirely to curriculum development, implementation, teaching, evaluation, and educational research. He conceived and implemented "Focal Problems," the first major commitment to early, integrated, problem-based learning in any medical school. With Dr. Tom Johnson, he also organized the four primary clinical teaching campuses for the College of Human Medicine, carried out (basic science/clinical science) faculty development, and later co-led the development of the upper peninsula program—a module for medical education in the rural setting. While at the Center for Educational Development, University of Illinois, Chicago, he participated in the clerkship study led by Dr. Engel. He was then commissioned by the Association of American Medical Colleges to organize and manage an interview study of student reactions to the first two years of medical school. Since the mid-1980s, his clinical work has been in addiction medicine. He has led numerous workshops and support groups for physicians, medical students, and other health care professionals on personal and professional coping and emotional and spiritual growth and development. Throughout his career, Dr. Ways has championed prevention and health maintenance. In recent years, he has founded and worked on Conscious Parenting, an enterprise devoted to formulating a set of "Prime Principles of Parenting," conducting workshops for parenting educators and physicians, and developing a set of assessments and operating principles for detecting and resolving problems in affective parenting at different stages of child development. He has gained additional perspectives on the vicissitudes and rewards of the medical education process by supporting the progress and careers of three daughters, all physicians. Dr. Ways is based in Seattle, where he consults in parenting, health promotion, and educational change. He is Visiting Professor of Medical Education at Northeastern Ohio Universities College of Medicine.

Dr. John D. Engel, trained as a social psychologist, has spent the majority of his professional career as a medical educator. He has been a pioneer in the definition and effective use of qualitative research paradigms in medical education. While he was on the faculty at the Center for Educational Development, he directed a qualitative phenomenological portrayal of the clinical clerkship in which six observers (including Dr. Ways and himself) were paired with medical students and spent over 500 hours in direct observation of clerkship activities. The rich and intricate culture of the clerkship, including its shadow side, was revealed in intimate detail. He has been principal investigator for many other studies of medical education and process. He is also the architect and founder of the University of Delaware-Jefferson Medical College integrated program wherein a student is accepted for premed with the understanding that if courses are completed satisfactorily, medical school admission is guaranteed without further application. The program is rich in behavioral science material. Currently, Dr. Engel is Vice President for Academic Affairs and Executive Associate Dean of Northeastern Ohio Universities College of Medicine.

Dr. Peter Finkelstein attended Michigan State University's College of Human Medicine when it was still in its formative stages and experienced much of the excitement and frustration of a clinical training experience that pioneered the community-based paradigm, with increased emphasis on the outpatient experience. His interest in the anatomy lab grew out of his own experience as a medical student. While a psychiatry resident and fellow at Stanford, he conducted a five-year study of the anatomy lab. He did 300 hours of direct observation and interviewing in an unparalleled study of student affect, reactions, and adaptations to working month after month with cadavers. This work has furnished a number of important insights as to how the preclinical experience influences the ways in which students approach and function (personally and professionally) in their clinical rotations. Dr. Finkelstein practices psychiatry in Woodside, CA. He also regularly coaches and consults with troubled corporate leadership.